HERBAL MAGICK

THE WEISER CONCISE GUIDE SERIES

HERBAL MAGICK

JUDITH HAWKINS-TILLIRSON

INTRODUCED BY
NANCY WASSERMAN

EDITED BY
NANCY AND JAMES WASSERMAN

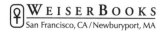
WEISERBOOKS
San Francisco, CA / Newburyport, MA

First published in 2007 by
Red Wheel/Weiser, LLC
With offices at:
500 Third Street, Suite 230
San Francisco, CA 94107
www.redwheelweiser.com

ISBN-10: 1-57863-411-3
ISBN-13: 978-1-57863-411-8

Library of Congress Cataloging-in-Publication Data

Hawkins-Tillirson, Judith.
The Weiser concise guide to herbal magick / by Judith Hawkins-
Tillirson ; introduced by Nancy Wasserman ; edited by Nancy and James
Wasserman.
    p. cm.
Includes bibliographical references.
ISBN 1-57863-411-3 (alk. paper)
1. Witchcraft. 2. Magic. 3. Herbs--Miscellanea.
I. Wasserman, Nancy. II. Wasserman, James, 1948- III. Title.
BF1572.P43H39 2007
133.4'3--dc22

                                            2007020347

Cover design by Maija Tollefson
Text design by Studio 31
Typeset in Adobe Sabon
Cover photograph © Visual Language

Printed in Canada

TCP

10 9 8 7 6 5 4 3 2 1

CONTENTS

Acknowledgments

I wish to thank Lord Hermes, *sine qua non.*

I wish to honor the memories of my mother, Martha Long Hawkins; my sister, Martha Hawkins Bigham; and my ex-husband and always friend, Patrick Michael Gaffney, who ever encouraged my writing. *Let us meet—know—remember—and love again.*

I wish to express boundless gratitude to two extraordinary teachers of O'Keefe High School: Jane Hatcher, who proved that History was not only alive, but exciting; and Pat Thornton, teacher of English, Italian, and French, who, with her husband Leon Thornton, has remained ever my friend and Muse, inspirational source *dulce et utile.*

I wish to thank my dear friends Richard Patz, Matthew Quellas, Lon Milo DuQuette, and Dr. Robert Wang for their continued friendship, esteem, encouragement, and generosity.

I wish to thank my employer, New Leaf Distributing, in the persons of my friends and bosses, Alim Thompson and Karen Price, for their support in my life in general and particularly while I was writing this work.

I wish upon my editors, Nancy and James Wasserman—my own personal Maat and Thoth—all the pleasures of boundless good karma for their unqualified patience, and for making me write this book.

I want to acknowledge Franca Gallo (of Merkur Publishing), Lisa-Marie Jackson (White Witch of Angelfire), and Jennifer Rose Emick (editor of About.com's Alternative Religions pages) for their generosity in allowing me to use materials under their care.

I wish to thank my beloved husband, Joseph Tillirson, who, before this project, had only *dreamed* he'd put up with a lot from a wife. You're right—you *do* love me the most!

And, finally, I'd like to give credit to my black-and-white tuxedo boy, polydactylic Feline-American, Harvey (brother of Ellwood P. Dowd), but one manifestation of Mercury, Trickster, Wily One, and Defeater of Locks, who has overseen in the most direct physical means possible the research, writing, and production of this work.

Any faults, errors, or misconceptions in this work are mine alone!

DEDICATION

To Nairn Galvin, Teacher of Herbs and all else.

"I am the soundless, boundless, bitter sea;
All things in the end shall come to me.
Mine is the kingdom of Persephone.
The inner earth, where lead the pathways three.
Who drinks the waters of that hidden well
Shall see the things whereof he dare not tell
Shall tread the shadowy path that leads to me
Diana of the Ways and Hecate,
Selena of the Moon, Persephone."

—Dion Fortune, **The Sea Priestess**

Introduction

I first met Judith Hawkins-Tillirson in 1988 when I attended my initial publishing-industry trade show. I was standing in the center of the American Booksellers Association Convention (now called Book Expo of America) in a trance—I had just been diagnosed with Lyme disease and was experiencing a raging fever. The bustle and bump of the convention floor whirled about me—it was nauseatingly surreal and I felt as if I were floating about six inches off the floor. Suddenly, a gentle voice pulled me back into "normal" consciousness: "Hi, my name is Judith. I'm so pleased to meet you." I focused in on a pair of warm brown eyes and knew immediately that this was "kin."

Throughout the course of the convention, we had the opportunity to spend some quality moments together. She recommended arnica to ease the pain in my joints and Rescue Remedy to ease the mental tension of being ill in a public venue. I followed her advice and managed to accomplish a great deal in a very stressful situation. During our time together, I found her to be a delightful ally and profoundly knowledgeable in both magick and herbalism. We have been fortunate enough to remain friends. I am often startled by her exceptional perceptions of events and situations. She has a well-rounded experience of, and appreciation for, not only the magick of herbs and potions, but high ceremonial magick and ritual. Her sense of humor is often a lifesaver in the sea of outrageous pomposity that surrounds and occasionally floods the occult environment. These delightful traits and skills run through every page of this book.

Judith's wisdom spans the broad spectrum of scholarship required of any serious occultist. Indeed, it is of utmost importance for any person on the Western path to have a well-rounded approach to all of the steps on the journey. One's knowledge base should include the study of herbalism. Despite the fact that it is a formidable weapon in the magical armory, herbalism is often neglected by ceremonial magicians. I think this is because some magicians feel the practice is too closely tied to what they consider "earth-based" religions—witchcraft, Druidism, or any of the varieties of modern Paganism—with no part to play in "high magick." This is a pity, because there is much to be gained from working with herbs. They are potent receptacles of their corresponding planets' energies. Occultists would do well to remember the lessons gleaned from the mage Cornelius Agrippa: Reach out and touch just one link of the Great Chain of Being and "the whole doth presently shake." Magicians who persist in the study of herbalism will cultivate a tool that can assist them to achieve the loftiest goals.

On the other hand, many witches and pagans tend to ignore the Qabala, thinking it is unbearably turgid, based in what they perceive as "Old Testament" principles. Judith takes a very practical approach to its use, pointing out and demonstrating its virtues as a boundless filing system. She lays out *The Weiser Concise Guide to Herbal Magick* using column XXXIX of 777 as a springboard for discussing the energies of plants and their corresponding planetary and astrological influences. This provides a great introduction to both herbalism and Qabala. Occultists who build proficiency in this relatively simple skill will expand their perception of the magical universe exponentially and increase the efficiency of their Great Work. Judith offers a practical approach to magical herbalism, regardless of your persuasion.

The Weiser Concise Guide to Herbal Magick explores the history and uses of herbs as well as their corresponding planetary and zodiacal energies. It provides clear instructions on their practical application, and even includes a chapter devoted to Franz Bardon's fluid condensers.

Take some time to enjoy and learn here. Even if you don't have the time or space to create a magical garden, Judith provides practical ways of working with herbs and their energies. Herbalism is sensual and meditative, providing a way of grounding your rituals (pardon the pun) and ensuring that you engage all aspects of your being in your magical practices. It is my hope that you enjoy this book as much as I have.

As always, best of luck to you in your magical endeavors.

Nancy Wasserman
New York City
Spring Equinox, 2007 e.v.

EDITORS' NOTE:

777 is mentioned as the basis of the herbal correspondences listed in the text of *The Weiser Concise Guide to Herbal Magick*. 777 was originally published by Aleister Crowley in 1909, revised and expanded in 1955, and later reprinted by Weiser. It is now available as *777 and Other Qabalistic Writings*, edited and introduced by Israel Regardie, also published by Weiser. It is acknowledged by all that the Golden Dawn correspondences as developed by S. L. MacGregor Mathers and others was the basis for the text, and that Crowley's friend and mentor, the adept Allan Bennett, also contributed to the editorial work of the initial publication.

777 was published before Crowley had fully come to grips with the message of *Liber AL vel Legis, The Book of the Law* (also available from Weiser). Verse 57 of chapter 1 states, in part: "All these old letters of my Book are aright; but צ is not the Star. This also is secret: my prophet shall reveal it to the wise." Crowley later switched the attributions of Tzaddi and Heh, the Star and the Emperor cards of the tarot, and the astrological attributions of paths 15 and 28 of the Tree of Life.

The tables in *777*, as published, list path 15 as Aries and path 28 as Aquarius. This is now understood to be path 15 as Aquarius and path 28 as Aries. Our text has been updated to reflect the "switch," as outlined in *The Book of the Law*. Thus we have modified the Tree of Life diagram, the Tables of Correspondences, and the attributions listed in the text.

This important issue of Thelemic doctrine may be studied further in *The Book of Thoth*, and *Magick, Liber ABA*, both by Aleister Crowley and both published by Weiser.

—NW and JW

FOREWORD

The Instruction of a magician, and what manner of man a Magician ought to be. This is what is required to instruct a *Magician* ... [It] is required of him, that he be a *Herbalist*, not only to be able to discern common *Simples*, but very skillful and sharp-sighted in the nature of all plants; for the uncertain names of plants, and their near likeness of one to another ... has put us to much trouble in some of our works and experiments. And as there is no greater inconvenience to any artificer, than not to know his tools that he must work with; so the knowledge of plants is so necessary to this profession, that indeed it is all in all.

—*Giambattista della Porta,* **Natural Magic**

Why do we need yet another magical herbal? It seems to me that as the world around us speeds up, we—who should, of all people, be sensitive to and aligned with cosmic rhythms—are as prone as anyone to being caught up in today's net of distractions. However, any gardener will tell you that there is no undertaking that teaches you more about being here now and being attuned to the life of the planet than working with plants.

There are dozens of magical herbals available; we all know this. I wanted to offer something different, something new, something besides the lists of magical herbs derived from the admittedly great Nicholas Culpeper and his teacher-mentor, John Lilly. If Renaissance herbalism or Astrology is not for you, you will find Culpeper's old works made new again by Mrs. Grieve's incalculable *Modern Herbal*. Without Lilly and Culpeper, we'd be very hard-put indeed to pick any *useful* herbal material out of the old grimoires. These two were among the very brave occultists who walked the thin line between the Hermetic and the heretical, during a time when straying an inch off that path meant certain death of a particularly unpleasant sort. We owe them an unimaginable debt. The planetary and astrological associations for the herbs and plants they give remain true and comprise much of the substance of magical herbalism today. These attributions did not just happen, however, and it's doubtful that a podcast from the gnomes informed us that they just *love* patchouli. One thing I'd like to do in

Key Scale	Hebrew Name of Numbers and Letters	Zodiacal and Elemental Attributions	Astro Symbols	COLUMN XXXIX OF 777 Plants, Real and Imaginary (Paths 15 and 28 revised)
1	Kether	Primum Mobile		Almond in Flower
2	Chokmah	Zodiac		Amaranth
3	Binah	Saturn	♄	Cypress, Opium Poppy
4	Chesed	Jupiter	♃	Olive, Shamrock
5	Geburah	Mars	♂	Oak, Nux Vomica, Nettle
6	Tiphareth	Sun	☉	Acacia, Bay, Laurel, Vine
7	Netzach	Venus	♀	Rose
8	Hod	Mercury	☿	Moly, Analonium Lewinii
9	Yesod	Moon	☽	[Banyan], Mandrake, Damiana
10	Malkuth	Elements		Willow, Lily, Ivy
11	Aleph	Air	△	Aspen
12	Beth	Mercury	☿	Vervain, Herb Mercury, Marjoram, Palm
13	Gimel	Moon	☽	Almond, Mugwort, Hazel as ☽, Ranunculus
14	Daleth	Venus	♀	Myrtle, Rose, Clover
15	Heh	Aquarius	♒	[Olive], Coconut
16	Vau	Taurus	♉	Mallow
17	Zain	Gemini	♊	Hybrids, Orchids
18	Cheth	Cancer	♋	Lotus
19	Teth	Leo	♌	Sunflower
20	Yod	Virgo	♍	Snowdrop, Lily, Narcissus
21	Kaph	Jupiter	♃	Hyssop, Oak, Poplar, Fig
22	Lamed	Libra	♎	Aloe
23	Mem	Water	▽	Lotus, all Water Plants
24	Nun	Scorpio	♏	Cactus
25	Samekh	Sagittarius	♐	Rush
26	Ayin	Capricorn	♑	Indian Hemp, Orchis Root, Thistle
27	Pé	Mars	♂	Absinthe, Rue
28	Tzaddi	Aries	♈	Tiger Lily, Geranium
29	Qoph	Pisces	♓	Unicellular Organisms, Opium
30	Resh	Sun	☉	Sunflower, Laurel, Heliotrope
31	Shin	Fire	△	Red Poppy, Hibiscus, Nettle
32	Tau	Saturn	♄	Ash, Cypress, Hellebore, Yew, Nightshade
32 bis		Earth	▽	Oak, Ivy
31 bis		Spirit	⊕	Almond in Flower

this magical herbal is to give a little history and context for this discipline. If I'm lucky, some drops of knowledge distilled from the great teachers of the past will splatter from history's cauldron and impart to us, if not wisdom, at least discrimination.

As critical and necessary as Lady Discrimination is, I do have another and even more pressing need for writing this small book on herbal magick, and that is to impart this claim:

Any magician who needs knowledge regarding the understanding and use of herbs in magick, will find absolutely everything in Column XXXIX, "Plants, real and imaginary," of Aleister Crowley's 777.

Please note: this material did not originate with Crowley; it was part of the magical curriculum of the Golden Dawn, which Crowley published in sundry ways after he left the Order. The core of the material did not even originate with the Golden Dawn, but was, I discovered, an echo of a ghost: not cohesive enough to be labeled "lore," yet undeniably a tendril of magical herb teaching that snaked its way through ancient works of materia medica, grimoires, and astrological correspondences until it flowered in the works of Éliphas Lévi. Lévi's works were so beloved by S. L. MacGregor Mathers, William Wynn Westcott, and the others of the Order that practically the whole of his writings were incorporated into its teaching materials in some form or another. Lévi was a profound student of Qabala, as well as a magical historian with knowledge as wide as it was deep. It was Lévi who took the few pieces of herb lore proven Qabalistically sound and incorporated them into a series of daily planetary magical workings to rival in intent even the sublime suggestions of the Renaissance philosopher and astrologer Marsilio Ficino.

What I'm trying to convey is: Column XXXIX of 777 is all you need to work herbal magick. Literally. You don't have to study the tables of correspondences to the 32 paths of the Tree of Life, learn Hebrew, undertake the Abramelin Working, spell "Kamea" (much less make one), or attempt any other discipline perhaps distasteful to the garden-variety witch or pagan simply to make use of it. It will save you so much time, and lend such a depth to your magical work that you'll wonder why you fought so hard against it. As far as you ritual magicians go—yeah, you guys, you know who you are—there's a lot more to Crowley and his teachers (yes, his teachers!) than you may have thought. He did not pop into this dimension fully informed, and he worked hard for the knowledge he imparted to his magical heirs. He thought herbal correspondences were important enough to merit their own column in *777*; and maybe you should, too.

To return to "discrimination," it has become even more precious since the burgeoning Internet has provided anyone with access to more instant information and disinformation than ever thought possible. However, as useful as the Internet is, information derived from it must be taken with bags, not grains, of salt. For instance: Sybil Leek, that dear and gnarly old hedgewitch, must be spinning in her grave at the web pages attributing to her what are actually crudely condensed instructions for the creation of elemental fluid condensers. The magical technology of the fluid condensers was solely a product of that great occult singularity, Franz Bardon. Why post it online (on more than a few sites) and claim it to be Lady Sybil's? Not only is it just wrong; it's so absolutely *unnecessary*. That's what I mean by "discrimination."

You don't need to know much, if any, Astrology or Qabala to benefit from this book, but I hope that something here inspires you to incorporate into your magical life some of the basics of these two very useful occult sciences. Your practices, and your life, will be so very much the richer for it. If you're a witch or pagan who thought the Qabala was too, well, *biblical* to be of any use whatever to you, I hope by the time you end your visit here you'll have changed your mind. It's a filing system, and will provide you with the single most convenient magical tool you'll ever encounter. Give it a try! It's another tool to help you refine your own Great Work; and, in the end, this is solely what the practice of magick is about.

Judith Hawkins-Tillirson
Sunday August 13, 2006 C.E.
Festival of Hecate

An Alarmingly Brief History
of Herbal Magick

When did the lemons learn
The same creed as the sun?
When did the smoke learn how to fly?
When do roots talk with each other?

—PABLO NERUDA, "Flies Enter a Closed Mouth"

The history of herbal magick is in equal parts fascinating, demanding, and aggravatingly frustrating. Fascinating because to research the subject is to begin to live with it, to follow the shoots and offshoots, to see its spread as it naturalizes normally in one geographical area, cultural milieu, or time period, but throws off odd, if not downright disturbing, sports[1] in another. Demanding because, beyond the mere historical timeline, serious students soon find themselves drawn inexorably into the more perverse aspects of herbal magick, e.g., the development of the notion of the four humors that has so central a role in so many antique occult disciplines—Astrology, alchemy, healing, and, of course, herbalism itself. Frustrating because researchers discover that, the deeper they dive into the subject, the murkier and darker the water becomes, until their initial effort to bring light is perforce abandoned. This is not to suggest that we shouldn't even start; it is, after all, the journey, not the arrival, that is more important, and we will become more knowledgeable magicians for the effort.

The one fundamental and critically important postulate in the study of herbal magick is our beloved formula from the Emerald Table of Hermes Trismegistus, elegantly phrased:

> *It is true and no lie, certain, and to be depended upon,*
> *that the superior agrees with the inferior, and the inferior*
> *with the superior, to the glory of the one thing.*

This tenet is the foundation for each and every occult discipline. Period. Although its earliest textual appearance can only be dated to *c.* 800 C.E., we find the same idea expressed by Plato in the Theory of Forms. Plato's theory, crudely simplified, states that there is in the divine realm an archetype or "form" for everything existing in the physical realm; the things of this Earth have their being only as instantiations of their form, or by participation in that form. This philosophical approach waned through the centuries, until it was revived by the Neoplatonists, who took that ball and ran it into a whole other court. We find that the entire *Corpus Hermeticum* is late antiquity's densely saturated, intellectually sophisticated, and magically erudite Neoplatonic stew.

As it happens, this savory and complex broth was, at the outset, a "stone soup" to which many profound and recondite thinkers added a turnip here, an onion there, a handful of parsley, simmer 600 or so years and bing! It went something like this: the Pre-Socratics and later the Stoics offered us their arguments detailing the four elements and suggesting the fifth, or quintessence—*Nous* or mind—now identified with spirit. At an early but unknown point, the four elements became linked in some ways with Hellenistic medicine's primary diagnostic, the four humors. But good old Aristotle (d. 322 B.C.E.) nailed that alignment down for us.

Equally murky is the move from the four elements of Hippocrates to the four elements of Astrology. Marilynn Lawrence writes:

> A Hippocratean would classify an individual's psychophysical nature into one of four types based on the qualities of hot, cold, moist, and dry. Astrologers borrowed and elaborated upon the psychology and character typology found in early medical theory ... In turn, Astrology in the Hellistic era was to ... inform medical theory.[2]

This occurred in four ways: physical type determined by the birth chart; iatromathematics (a $2 word if ever there was one), which considered auspicious and inauspicious times; the "sympathies and antipathies between healing plants and celestial bodies"; and the predictions of an illness' course.

The two disciplines of medicine and Astrology continued to bounce these ideas back and forth, developing them all the while, until the great Græco-Roman astrologers like Claudius Ptolemey, Manilius, and Vettius Valens presented the modern astrologer with an elemental arrangement that is almost recognizable as such. It is, however, that third way of sympathies and antipathies that concerns us the most, for it is here that herbal magick as we know it today has its inception.

What!? you ask. No unbroken line of herbal lore, no discernable lineage of herbal magical workings from antiquity until now? No. Sadly, no. The astrologer-priests of the world between the rivers Tigris and Euphrates, it is true, had developed, over some three or four millennia, a complex system relating certain gods to their specific plants and planets. And we have record upon record of their magical formulæ, spellwork, rituals, and liturgies. These would be of inestimable value to us if more than a scant handful of the actual plant species could be identified. Later, Chaldean mages like Ostanes (5th century B.C.E.), teacher of the Pseudo-Democritus, in turn purported teacher of "the more shadowy" Bolos of Mendes, are all central figures in the history of herbal magick. Bolos was alleged to have written a collection of books of magical lore, herbalism, and ritual instruction titled *Cheirokmeta*.[3] Although he is supposed to have gleaned this unbelievably ancient mystic and magical lore from the powerful magicians of Persia, Arabia, Ethiopia, and Egypt, all indications point rather to his wholesale plagiarism of an earlier work on magical plants by one Cleemporus.[4]

Ostanes is said to have introduced Persian magick into Greece, but if you think you're going to be able to pick up a thread of magical herbal tradition there, well, then, I have some "virgin" emeralds to sell you. At the folkloric level, the record of magical spells conducted with the benefit of herbs is impressive and ancient. The *Odyssey*, composed as early as the ninth century B.C.E., even has the god Hermes providing Odysseus with moly to thwart the potions and spells of "the goddess" Circe. Unfortunately, the multiple examples of Greek herb-based sympathetic magick show no system of agreement of plant to god, to part of the body, or to any recognizable methodology at all, save for the correspondences overlaid on the substances used by the magical worker.

Typical of these spells is the one satirically rendered by Theocritus (3rd century B.C.E.) in his *Idyll II: The Sorceress*, which concludes with the sorceress sending her maid with some unidentified flowers to knead (Cheirokmeta, remember?) over the cad's threshold while chanting: "I knead the bones of Delphis." An unsystematic mess, but, fueled by the sorceress' emotions, it was probably very effective, to Delphis' regret. Exciting—but is it helpful in detecting an identifiable discipline of herbal magick? Not as such. It does, however, offer an indication of why, in contemporary popular opinion, the magick of the root-cutters (*Rhyzotomia*—thickened root or "rhizome") dealt exclusively with "dark magick" and *pharmakas* (literally, "poisons").

Fast-forward through centuries of poor translations and thinly disguised plagiarism of the great *Materia Medica* of Dioscorides (*c.* 60 C.E.), augmented or not with material from Apuleius and Pliny the Elder, and we arrive finally in 1597 at the doorstep of modern herbalism with the *Herbal* of the botanist and physician John Gerard.

Gerard was the first herbalist to provide illustrations of the herbs under discussion that were drawn from observation of the living plants. This one step meant that, for the first time in history, readers had a field guide that accurately portrayed the plants. Without, say, any little breasts that earlier tended to show up on drawings of a "female" mandrake root, for instance. However, Gerard set out to demythologize herbal lore and, throughout the thousand-plus pages of his *Herbal,* we find him heaping the kind of abuse of magical considerations that we encountered in Pliny—while still employing, of course, the methodology of the Four Humors. Gerard is, therefore, a necessary, but not sufficient, source for modern herbal magick.

For this, we turn instead to Nicholas Culpeper—astrologer, physician, herbalist, populist—the great leveler who single-handedly broke the stranglehold on medical knowledge held by the Royal College of Physicians. In 1649, he published his English translation of their precious *Pharmacopoeia Londonensis,* now titled the *London Physical Directory*, thus empowering the literate populace of England to doctor themselves.

There's so much more that is sadly outside the scope of these few pages. We are unable to treat the Doctrine of Signatures, suggested in the *Zohar,* defined by Paracelsus, promoted by Giambattista della Porta, and surprisingly revived in the works of Samuel Hahnemann, Dr. Edward Bach, and Franz Bardon. Central to the Doctrine of Signatures is that the Great Maker placed a "sign," or signature, on each medical plant indicating the body part, if not the actual malady, that plant was created to treat—a familiar example is the spotted, "lung-shaped" leaves of the *Pulmonaria* or lungwort, used for centuries in treating lung disorders.

I will also spare you the torturous (and, candidly, pathological) wading through centuries of the old grimoires, laboriously tracing which plants differed in planetary attributions from the *Kyranides* to the *Picatrix,* through Al-Biruni's *Tahfim* to Albertus Magnus' *Book of Secrets.* By the time we arrive happily (if breathlessly) at Agrippa in the 16th century and William Lilly in the 17th, the planetary-herb attributions have begun to shape up and we can see where and how Lévi derived the core of his plant assignments.

Let us now turn to Israel Regardie and Dion Fortune, the 20th-century occultists to whom we owe so very much. Associated with the Golden Dawn (G∴D∴) at two different times, they did not meet until 1932, some months after Regardie published both his *Tree of Life* and *A Garden of Pomegranates.* There's a letter from Fortune, who had been sent a copy of each book, to Regardie dated November

1 of that year. She writes the author that she thinks "very highly of both the books, and especially *The Tree of Life*. Of *A Garden of Pomegranates*":

> I judge from the correspondences given in *The Garden of Pomegranates*, that you are using the old Golden Dawn System, which is the one I use myself. I think it is far and away the best. Crowley gives it away in 777, but I have also got the Mathers MSS to check it by.[5]

With a few minor exceptions, Regardie's attributions in *The Garden of Pomegranates* closely follow those of Crowley in 777. Regardie, however, limits himself to the one plant he considers most important to each path's central symbolism.

Just a very few more notes before we start climbing down the Tree.

Please note that for the purpose of this book I consider every instance on the Tree of a specific energy to be equivalent to and interchangeable with every other occurrence of that energy.[6] For example, Mars energy is Mars energy, whether we encounter it at Geburah/fifth sephira as the Realm of Mars, or on path 28 as Aries, or as path 24's Scorpio (both ruled by Mars), or on path 27 as Mars the planetary member of our solar system. Further, fiery Mars lends that energy to the plants of the element of Fire. Further, note that five of the seven planets rule two signs each, while the Sun and Moon, the Luminaries, rule only Leo and Cancer respectively.

Moon—Cancer
Mercury—Gemini and Virgo
Venus—Taurus and Libra
Sun—Leo
Mars—Aries and Scorpio
Jupiter—Sagittarius and Pisces
Saturn—Capricorn and Aquarius

(This is classical Astrology; we have no time to waste on those Johnny-come-lately, fly-by-night planets Uranus, Neptune, and Pluto. And the Earth's in the center of the solar system, just so's you know!)

Finally, I use the words "herb" and "plant" interchangeably.

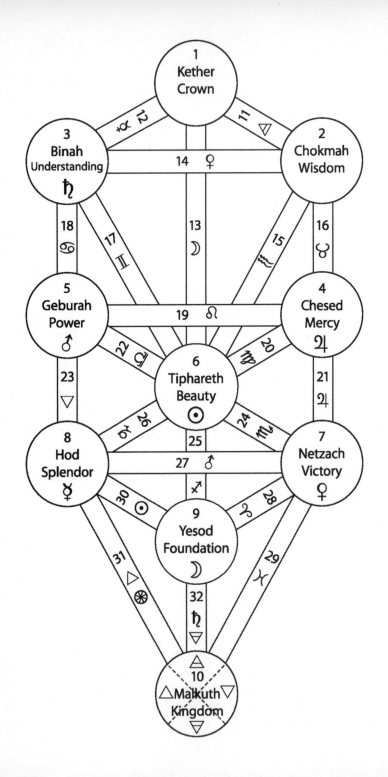

PART ONE:

The Planetary Correspondences of Herbal Magick

✳

Chapter One

THE PLANTS OF SATURN

Binah: Cypress, Opium Poppy
26th Path, Capricorn: Indian Hemp, Orchis Root, Thistle
15th Path, Aquarius: [Olive], Coconut
32nd Path, Saturn: Ash, Cypress, Hellebores, Yew, Nightshade

"Nobody slides, my friend." —Willie Nelson

In classical Astrology, Saturn is the most difficult planet for the average person to experience. He demands maturity and responsibility—aspects of living that are the least fun in a chart or a life. Saturn is considered the Great Teacher by astrologers. We are urged to accept his lessons with as much grace and gratitude as we can muster, and to learn to evolve spiritually from the experiences he brings. At the very least, we should be able to stop going through the same challenges time and time again whenever Saturn in our chart is activated by transit or progression. Kronos, the father of Zeus, is confused in name with the Greek word for time, "chronos." So Kronos came to be Old Father Time, with his hourglass and sickle—the Grim Reaper. Ruling old things, antiques, immovable property (real estate), governments, bones, teeth, and particularly the knees (the skeleton and support of the body or the shell, the protector of it), Kronos can seem to personify the cliché "death and taxes," the only sure things in life.

The mythological associations are with the Titan Kronos, the youngest and strongest of Gaia's children, the only one willing to undertake the castration of their father, Uranus, so that Gaia's children could be born. However, Saturn also banished everything threatening. Kronos (Saturn) concerned himself with his own security, with self-preservation, with assuring his sphere of absolute influence. He did not look kindly to the future. Anything new appeared suspect.

There's the ruler of Capricorn we all know and love! To the ancient Greeks, Kronos was an influence bringing peace and introspection. Marsilio Ficino, the great Renaissance philosopher, finds Saturn to be of the greatest utility. He writes, in his *Three Books on Life:*

> The contemplating intellect ... exposes itself somewhat to Saturn. To this faculty alone is Saturn propitious.... For Saturn has relinquished the ordinary life to Jupiter; but he claims for himself a life sequestered and divine. To the minds of those who are truly sequestered as much as possible, he is in a way friendly, as to his kinfolk.[1]

In other words, to those devoted to the interior life, Saturn is a benefactor. Crowley writes of those whose maturity, chronological and spiritual, puts them under Saturn's reign:

> Life is to them a religion of which they are the priests, an eternal sacrament of which perhaps the ecstasy is dulled, but which they consume with ever-increasing reverence. Joy and sorrow have been balanced, and the tale thereof is holy calm.[2]

This theme, however, is stated by philosophers who can look at the highest expression of Saturn. Lévi, on the other hand, writes that the magical works of Saturn are the "works of malediction and death."[3]

The Plants of Binah: The Sphere of Saturn
Cypress, Opium Poppy

Saturn's energies are found in paths 3, 15, 26, and 32; these plants are the ones employed in all his magical works, so let us turn to the plants given in 777 for these paths. Crowley writes:

> The Cypress pertains to Saturn. The Opium Poppy is connected with sleep, night and understanding.

Cypress: Cypress traditionally grows in cemeteries. In ancient Greece, it was a tree sacred to Hades, Lord of the Underworld. Culpeper writes of the cypress:

This tree is under the government of Saturn. The cones or nuts are mostly used, the leaves but seldom; they are accounted very drying and binding, good to stop fluxes of all kinds ...; they prevent the bleeding of the gums, and fasten loose teeth.... [4]

Remember: Saturn binds, dries, and brings to a stop.

Cypress (*Cupressus sempervirens*) can live to a very great age. Wood cut from it, Theophrastus notes, is the least likely to decay.

Opium Poppy: The opium poppy (*Papaver somniferum*) is almost too notorious to discuss. It is an ancient symbol of Persephone, Hades' consort and Queen of the Dead. The shape of the poppy's seedpod is that of Persephone's other famous plant, the pomegranate. They are iconographically identical. Recall that Saturn's energies are aligned with the realms of the dead; further, using the opium poppy medicinally or recreationally stops pain, slows the body, and constipates. No plant has provided more utility than the opium poppy, nor is any more abused. *Potter's Therapeutics, Materia Medica and Pharmacy* describes opium as:

> ... an analgesic, hypnotic, antispasmodic, diaphoretic and narcotic. It first stimulates and afterwards depresses the cerebrum, heart and respiratory apparatus, and ... it kills by paralyzing the respiratory centres in the medulla. It stops the patient from sensing pain, it stops peristalsis, and an overdose will stop the breath.[5]

The stimulation of the cerebrum, as well as the mental abstractions provided by its use, support Crowley's characterization of "Understanding," the translation of "Binah." These mental actions are certainly circumscribed by Ficino's "contemplating intellect."

The 26th Path: Capricorn
Indian Hemp, Orchis Root, Thistle

Of these, Crowley writes: "Thistle is hard, stubborn and spiky. Orchis Root is connected with the Cult of Pan. Indian Hemp is tough and fibrous, thus used for making ropes ... " For bindings? Thistle is also a tough and fiercely self-protective plant. It is opportunistically invasive to the detriment of native species, as birds scatter its seeds across wide areas; it grows happily in the smallest, poorest, rockiest crevice. Orchis root, which is nothing but the root of the orchid, is on this list because of its resemblance to the male genitalia or parts thereof; in fact, the Greek word ορχιζ (orchis) means testicle, bringing to mind Kronos' castration of his father, Uranus. A further connection is found in the equally ancient name for orchis root, satyrion, that is, satyr's root, named for those lust-driven half-goat beings. In other words, orchis root/satyrion signifies a horny old goat, which is rather what is portrayed in the tarot card belonging to this path, The Devil. We will encounter this plant again on the 17th path.

The 15th Path: Aquarius
[Olive], Coconut

For Saturn's other sign, Aquarius, we find listed olive (bracketed, to be sure) and coconut. Crowley doesn't give us any comment on olive, and any comment I may make on coconut would be as far-fetched as his own remark:

> Cocoanut: this attribution is doubtful. There may be some connection with Juno as giving milk or with the symbol of the Waterbearer, because the tree gives us fruit from the air.[6]

Or—and perhaps this is due to my just having completed research on orchis/satyrion—maybe the husked nut in its hairy shell is as evocative of a testicle as satyrion root. The rulership of Aquarius had been assigned to the "recently discovered" Uranus—for two centuries at least—and we're back to the castration of Uranus by his son, Kronos. One final and curious connection of coconut to Saturn, rather laterally through the opium poppy of Binah, is this: in the book *The Seven Sisters of Sleep* (first published 1860), the author describes the most common form of taking opium in Southeast Asia as using a water pipe made from a coconut shell.

The 32nd Path: Saturn
Ash, Cypress, Hellebores, Yew, Nightshade

Ash: Crowley writes:

> Ash is given in connection with the phrase, "ashen pale." (The real nature of the tree is more properly Solar.) In other cases, in connection with the ideas of death, melancholy, poison, etc.[7]

The ash was given to Saturn by Lévi. This appears odd, since this tree is one that loves sunlight, grows straight and tall, and, Hageneder writes:

> contains the best qualities of the most different trees: soft and firm; fast and persistent; graceful and strong; linear and round. A German saying calls Oak the King, and the Ash the high king among trees.[8]

Poor old crabbed, cramped Saturn gives few of these qualities, except perhaps firmness and persistence. However, I believe that we can find another association for ash that relates to the planet of the 32nd path. For one thing, the ash is male, female, or hermaphroditic, with male, female, and hermaphroditic flowers on the same tree. The tarot card given to the 32nd path is XXI, The Universe. In *The Book of Thoth*, Crowley writes of this card:

> Saturn, therefore, is masculine; he is the old god, the god of fertility, the sun in the south; but equally, the Great Sea, the great Mother . . . [9]

Yew: Like cypress, yew is a traditional cemetery tree, and is also noted for its extreme longevity. Some of the yews found in English church-yards are 4000 years old—proof, Steve Blamires writes in *Celtic Tree Mysteries*, that the churches were deliberately raised near to an already ancient tree. Robert Graves calls yew "the death-tree in all European countries, sacred to Hecate in Greece and Italy." It shares, with the boxwood, the distinction of having the hardest wood of any tree in the European temperate zone. Yew is renowned as the wood that made the best bows. We can speculate that the yew of Saturn's 32nd path provides the wood for Diana's bow at Yesod (and the 25th path).

That the yew lacks resin ("juice") is one reason it is not a true conifer. It is almost impossible to tell the age of a yew because it lives to such advanced years. When it does begin to die, it does so from the inside out, so that the rings that would indicate its age are destroyed. It is significant to consider that the new growth occurs within the shell of the old and even eventually takes over the original crown of the tree, making a young yew indistinguishable from an old one. By reason of this "immortality," many researchers find the yew, rather than the ash, to be Yggdrasil, the World Tree of the Norse sagas. The yew's longevity, and its toxicity, certainly earn it a place in the plants of Saturn.

There is one other curious aspect to the tree I'd like to mention in passing, related as well to the banyan, a tree of Luna. Yew is placed on the 32nd path, from Luna to Malkuth and Malkuth to Luna. Both the banyan and the yew are noted for their aerial "root" habits; branches or their offshoots grow downward to the ground, where they take root and form a new tree, eventually making dense colonies. I find in this fact a perfect consistency, presented botanically, with the actions of the Tree of Life; or, one may suggest, "phytology recapitulates ontology."

Hellebore: Hellebore (*Helleborus officianalis*) was used anciently and cautiously as a purgative, both of the body and of the mind. *Elein* is Greek for "to injure" and *bora* means "food." Pliny mentions the uses of the black and the white hellebore as insecticide, and as a poison for arrow tips. Leaving no stone, however fantastical, unturned, he gives his reader a list of conditions treated by hellebore that includes (among several others) insanity, white elephantiasis, and flatulence.

Culpeper notes that "since the Hellebore belongs to Saturn it is therefore no marvel if it has some sullen conditions with it, and would be far safer, being purified by the alchymist than given raw. Goat's milk is an antidote for it ... being beaten to powder, and strewed upon foul ulcers, it eats away the dead flesh, and instantly heals them: nay, it helps gangrenes in the beginning."[10]

Virtually the entire family is noted for toxic, burning, or drying qualities. The *Helleborus* family is closely related to the *Ranunculacae* (buttercups). Botanist Thomas Elpel, writing in *Botany in a Day*, calls this family

> ... a window back in time. If you travel back a hundred million years to see the first flowering plants you will find species similar to those of the Buttercup family today.... Of all the families of flowering plants, today's Buttercups and their allies ... have retained the most ancestral characteristics.[11]

There we have it: a primitive (i.e., old) plant family of a drying and poisonous disposition. Did I mention that hellebores prefer shady to sunny spots? That they bloom in the dead of winter around the time of the Saturnalia, untroubled by the cold, and that their blooms last for months? It's an altogether lovely ornamental plant, with glossy, evergreen leaves, growing in conditions of shade and dryness where few other plants will survive, let alone thrive and increase happily. *That's* a plant of Saturn!

Nightshade: The nightshade family comprises, at one end, some of the most useful and life-nourishing plants—the potato, tomato, capsicums (bell and chili peppers), eggplant, and lima bean—and some of the deadliest to human life, like henbane, belladonna, datura, and the mandrake. Tobacco is a member of the family, as is the petunia. Many of the plants have analgesic and sedative uses; others of the family will simply kill you. Some of them, prepared correctly, can cause hallucinations: famously, *Atropa Belladonna, Datura* (jimson/loco weed), *Hyoscamus niger* (henbane), and the *Mandragora off.* Some of these are ingredients in the classical Flying Ointment recipes of the witches, the use of any one of which is a means of "rising on the planes" that demands scrupulous attention to detail. We will be considering mandragora in more detail at Luna.

Chapter Two

THE PLANTS OF JUPITER

Chesed: Olive, Shamrock
21st Path, Jupiter: Hyssop, Oak, Poplar, Fig
25th Path, Sagittarius: Rush
29th Path, Pisces: Unicellular Organisms, Opium

"I was a free man in Paris ..." —Joni Mitchell

Jupiter's bailiwick ranges all the way from Sugar Daddy to Demiurgos. In Astrology, Jupiter is the Greater Benefic, bringer of all good things, protector of the weak, upholder of the Good. In *General Principles of Astrology*, Crowley writes:

> Zeus, or Jupiter, is more than lord of air. He is the heir of Saturn, and the father of the gods. In him is to be found the principle of human generation and the joy of life ... Blessings flock about his feet as dogs greet their master ... And here is danger—the danger of plethora. Even Jupiter may sit too long at the banquet ... It is important for each of us to emphasize the noble and the religious aspects of Jupiter. He is in a dangerous position between the leaden Saturn and the iron Mars.[1]

Jupiter is the planet given to higher education, to religion of an outward type (since his house, the 9th, sits at the top, i.e., the most public part, of the chart), and to philosophical speculation.

As lord of the planetary sphere of Chesed, we see him in the more exalted role of world creator, being the first sephirah encountered after the Abyss. Here, then, is found his role as Demiurge.

Lévi defines magical workings belonging to Jupiter, as "works of ambition and intrigue" best executed on a Thursday, "a day of great religious and political operations." The working should happen in his proper hours. Other appropriate works are anything involving luck or gambling, publishing, travel (long-distance), and large things. Since we're only concerned with the classical Astrology of the Qabala, Jupiter co-rules Sagittarius and Pisces—organized, outer, conventional religion, as well as the inner, far less formal, mystical sensibilities.

The Plants of Chesed: The Sphere of Jupiter
Olive, Shamrock

Crowley writes:

> The Olive is attributed to Jupiter because of its softness and richness.... The Shamrock of four leaves, a good-luck plant, suggests Jupiter. The Opium Poppy is Jupiterian as giving relief from pain, quiet, and olympian detachment.[2]

Olive: Hageneder finds, in the classification "virgin" applied to olive oil, a reference to the virgin goddess Athene, who is also connected to the olive because she bestowed the olive tree on the ancient Greeks. The oil is one of the most healthful ones for cooking and eating; monounsaturated and cholesterol-lowering, it protects the heart and aids digestion and liver function—not surprising, since Jupiter also rules that organ.

Olive oil is always the base of anointing oils, whether from the Hebrew, Christian, or Western Occult traditions, and is the traditional fuel for ritual lamps. Mrs. Grieve notes that in the Bible, Moses exempted from military service men who worked at cultivating the Olive, and that the victor in the Olympic games was crowned with its leaves.[3]

Shamrock: Crowley mentions the number four for Chesed, and "luck" for Jupiter. The "four-leaf clover" has come to be identified with the oxalis family and sold under names like "good-luck plant" and "lucky shamrock." Originally, the "four-leaf clover" was simply that, a white clover (*Trifolium repens*) with four leaves—a deviation or "sport" from the usual *Trifolium*; hence, you'd be lucky to find one. Since the clover is not dependable for producing four leaves, the oxalis became a substitute "shamrock," so that grocery stores could have something else to sell their customers in March.

The 21st Path: Jupiter
Hyssop, Oak, Poplar, Fig

Hyssop: The plants for this path show Jupiter in several different aspects. Crowley, or MacGregor Mathers, added hyssop to Lévi's original list in *Transcendental Magic*. Of hyssop, Crowley writes "[it] is Jupiterian on account of its religious use in lustration." Ritual

cleanliness is quite an important aspect of any ritual work; there are
several Old Testament references to a hyssop being used for asperging,
notably Psalms 51:7. In several other verses, it is paired with cedar.
The authors of *Plants of the Bible* mention that:

> ... even today in some Roman Catholic churches the brush used for
> sprinkling holy water is called a "hyssop."[4]

There has been extensive research and speculation about the
plant's true identity, but all agree on one point: the plant Linnaeus
named *Hyssopus officinalis* is not it. This plant is not native to the
Middle East.

> Unfortunately, the precise identification of this Biblical plant *ezov*
> is unquestionably the most puzzling and controversial of all the
> words in the Bible applying, or thought to apply, to plants and plant
> products.[5]

Does this botanical muddle concern the magical herbalist? Yes and
no. As a student of magical herbs, it always enhances your understanding to inform yourself to whatever degree possible about the
plants and herbs you are using in your magical operations. Deepened
understanding can only augment your work. Reflection on the herbs
"traditional" to each path will show you aspects of the Tree of Life
that may not have occurred to you before. The yew-banyan similarity
of aerial roots mentioned earlier, for instance, and the fact that these
plants are found on the 32nd and 9th paths respectively, suggests the
"rooting" of the Tree of Life in Malkuth, as well as the "tying" of
Malkuth to the Tree above it. That's the kind of "Aha!" moment a
study of plants will bring you.

However, magicians should also work with an eye to the prag-
matic. In this case, for instance, you'd never be able to make use of the
hyssop—a very useful herb, and one called for in numerous spells—in
a ritual or magical working, because you wouldn't know what the
actual thing was. I would never condone or suggest a haphazard
approach to magick, but herbal fundamentalism will not get you very
far in your particular Great Work. This is, I believe, one reason the
average magical or astrological herbal gives such long lists of plants for
each sign and planet—so that magicians or herbal practitioners are not
caught short, as it were.

My own solution, since I didn't know any better then, was to uti-
lize *Hyssopus off.* in my workings. It has, after all, been classified as

hyssop in the official Linnaean nomenclature for well over 250 years, and it has been used by magicians for centuries as the plant of Biblical fame that purges and makes clean. It has surely been suffused with this energy by now! Dion Fortune has some pertinent remarks on this point:

> Plants also we find credited with a varying degree of "psychic activity." The ancients had an elaborate system of attribution of plants to the different forms of subtle force. Some of these, of course, are fantastic, but there are certain broad principles which give guidance. Wherever we find a plant traditionally associated with any deity [or energy] we may be fairly certain that plant has been proven to have affinities with the type of force that deity represents.[6]

At this point, almost forty years after my first embarrassing attempts at ritual, I still use *Hyssopus off.* because I have come to understand that, regardless of all the props magicians have at their disposal, the most significant of the tools, and the only "real" ones, are their minds and their magical intention.

Oak: Crowley writes of the oak (*Quercus*) and poplar (*Populus*):

> The Oak is traditionally sacred to Jupiter, perhaps because it is the king of trees as Jupiter is king of the gods. The Poplar is given on account of its soft and easily swollen wood and because of its great height.[7]

According to Fred Hageneder in *The Meaning of Trees,* the oak was, in fact, associated with weather gods, particularly the thunder, sky, and lightning gods, across all the Indo-European cultures of Bronze Age Europe.

Of the several sky gods to whom the oak was sacred, Zeus, once merely the Greek god of lightning and later King of Olympus, is perhaps the most famous. The oracular oak in the grove at Dodona was a tree of prophecy and a cultic center of his early worship.

For invaluable information on the oak (and so much more!), please see Robert Graves' masterpiece *The White Goddess.*[8]

Poplar: The poplar's "soft and easily swollen wood" must refer to Jupiter's co-rulership of the watery Pisces. The second quality Crowley mentions, its great height, certainly earns poplar its place in this category.

Fig: The fig is an arresting addition to this list. Crowley suggests that "The Fig is Jupiterian because of its soft, swollen and, so to speak, sensual pulp; and also because of its rich purple colour, suggesting episcopal vestments."[9]

Crowley is correct in the fig/sensuality connection, as its split, ripened fruit has ever invoked the female genitalia. The fig is thus associated with Venus. But the god more properly aligned with the fig is Dionysus, who was titled *Philosykos*, "Friend of the Fig," in Attica because he brought that tree to Greece.

None of this helps us justify the fig in this Jupiterian list, however. Some more relevant associations are perhaps found in the fig tree's sometime identification as the Tree of Knowledge of Good and Evil of *Genesis*, or the Hebrew's association of the fig tree with peace, prosperity, and plenty (all Jupiterian concepts) as well as the Islamic notion of the Tree of Heaven (since the Prophet Mohammed swore by it).

The 25th Path: Sagittarius
Rush

The list for the 25th path, Sagittarius, is brief: rush, which Crowley notes "is used for making arrows." The term "rush" carries with it numerous possible significations, including grasses in general, papyrus, reeds, and the bulrushes of Mosaic fame. (I'm certain the fact that every Sagittarian I've ever known is always in a mad rush is total coincidence.) The bulrush, *Arundo donax,* or Persian reed, is a gigantic grass, growing from eight to eighteen feet tall. This plant was used for many purposes by the ancients—for walking sticks, fishing rods, measuring rods, and musical pipes—and is still today. I rather fancy this particular plant for the "rush" referred to in the magical alphabet, because it has so many associations that are Sagittarian or Jupiterian.

First, it is a huge plant, and Jupiter/Sagittarius rule big things. Second, it is a plant that grows in marshy places and along watersides. Think of the story of Moses being drawn from the water. Jupiter, Sagittarius' ruler, also co-rules Pisces, the most watery of the water signs. With Moses, we have both the icon of a religious leader (Jupiter), and a suggestion of the Temperance card of the tarot (Sagittarius), which, in most decks, has an angel standing with one foot on land and one in water. Finally, there is the fact that the use of the plant for walking sticks or canes aligns perfectly with the meaning of the Hebrew letter given to this path—*Samekh,* which means "prop" or "crutch." Lacking access to this plant, however, I feel that papyrus[10] or any waterside reed can be substituted in magical work.

The 29th Path: Pisces
Unicellular Organisms, Opium

For the 29th path, that of Pisces, the attributions include unicellular organisms and opium. Crowley writes:

> Opium is given because of its power to produce a peaceful dreamy condition which is liable to end in a stagnation of the mental faculties. Unicellular Organisms are possibly attributed here because they are so frequently found in pools.[11]

As far as this path goes, Crowley explains these two items fairly well. Opium should probably be referred to as the opium poppy, *Papaver somniferum,* since the discussion is of the plant form and not the drug. However, with the opium poppy, we will again remember Jupiter as the physician and lord of release.

Chapter Three

THE PLANTS OF MARS

Geburah: Oak, Nux Vomica, Nettle
28th Path, Aries: Tiger Lily, Geranium
24th Path, Scorpio: Cactus
27th Path, Mars: Absinthe, Rue

"Bring me my Broadsword and clear understanding ..."
—Jethro Tull

Mars is named by astrologers classical and modern as the "Lesser Malefic" (Saturn playing the Greater). He rules male energy and, more broadly, energy pure and simple—whether it's as passive as iron oxidation (producing the red rust found also in our blood, those precious little red corpuscles working to carry oxygen to the cells of our body) or as aggressive as the bombing of a city. The metal given to the planet Mars is iron. The ore is forged into steel for both the sword and the scalpel—Mars rules surgeons as well as soldiers.

Astrologer Ellynor Barz points out that Ares, the only son of Zeus and Hera, was a child unloved because he was rowdy, unruly, boisterous, and disobedient. His worship was neglected among humans until the time of Rome, where his protective nature was emphasized along with his warlike side. After Jupiter ("Greatest and Best"), the Romans considered him the most powerful god. How Ares translates into classical Astrology is shown by this typical description of a well- and ill-placed planet Mars penned in the 17th century by Jean-Baptiste Morin:

> Mars well placed. Brave, strong, spirited, noble, bold, arrogant, boastful ... full of contempt for other men, irascible ... eager for revenge, obeying no one ... eager for dominance, craving battles and conflicts, arrogant tyrants.
> ... Badly placed. Unscrupulous, unjust, pitiless, arrogant, quarrelsome, seditious, loud-mouthed, reckless, mad, cruel, assassins, murderers, tyrants, drunkards ...[1]

Sounds pretty dire for the Martian types, Arians and Scorpios. However, Greek mythology gives us some hope: while Mars and Venus sired children like Deimos (fear) and Phobos (terror), they also engendered Eros and Harmonia, who, according to Barz, was "[the] most beautiful daughter of Venus, in whom wildness, gentleness, desire and pleasure unite in perfect harmony."[2]

One can, therefore, suggest that the works of Mars, when guided by the loving hand of Venus, can be of a much more beneficial nature. In fact, some sources claim Mars was only at peace in her presence.

Magical workings belonging to Mars include acts of aggression, defensiveness, and counter-attacks. Protective magical work, particularly for those involved in wartime pursuits, also come under his aegis. Mars is the energy to contact to attain a successful outcome to a surgery. Needless to say, Mars is important energy to invoke when the magician is attempting to increase personal courage. Ficino wrote that "To offset timidity, at the first hour of Mars, with Scorpio rising[3] make images of Mars armed and crowned."[4]

The Plants of Geburah: The Sphere of Mars
Oak, Nux Vomica, Nettle

Crowley writes:

> The Oak and Hickory[5] are attributed here because of the hardness of their wood.... The Nettle, on account of its burning sting.... The Oak does have martial associations since among all cultures from ancient times until fairly recently, its tough wood was used in the construction of fortifications or battleships. [The] ancient Gauls and the Romans associated the oak with Mars Sylvanus, the god of agriculture and healing.[6]

Oak: In later Roman mythology, Mars was considered a pre-founder of Rome, siring Romulus and Remus by a vestal virgin. Hageneder finds Mars' influence on the oak to be primary when considered in the light of planetary rhythms on the flora of Earth. The astringent and drying properties of the oak's tannic acid do sit better with fiery Mars than with Jupiter's soft moistness. Finally, some oaks, due to their tremendous root systems and thick bark, are able to withstand even a forest fire.

Nux Vomica: For *Nux Vomica*, Crowley notes that it made Geburah's list:

... on account of its tonic properties and the action of strychnine in causing the contraction of muscles with convulsive violence.[7]

Daintily put. The small tree is poisonous in all its parts; the fruit has a smooth shell, horned internally, and contains five flat, circular seeds. Even the flowers, Mrs. Grieve says, have a "disagreeable smell." One notable element of strychnine is its unbelievably intense bitterness. *Potter's Therapeutics* notes that its presence is discernable in as little as one part per million. When Crowley was writing, it was used as a tonic and digestive aid. However, these days, it is most commonly used in its safest form, homeopathically. Even reading the most guarded account of strychnine poisoning gives me the screaming wimwams.

Nettle: Here's an honest herb of Mars, one whose effects last only a few minutes and are never fatal. *Urtica urens* is a feisty member of the mint family (always indicated by their square stems). The leaves resemble nothing so much as common catnip (*Nepeta cataria*) until it flowers with long tassels. You are well advised not to allow it access to any part of your unprotected skin, however. Mrs. Grieve writes that the entire plant is downy, and is also covered with stinging hairs. Each "hair" is a very sharp, polished hollow spine that arises from a swollen base that contains the venom, an acrid fluid, the active principle of which is bicarbonate of ammonia. When, in consequence of pressure, the sting pierces the skin, the venom is instantly expressed, causing irritation and inflammation.

Not only is this plant an arsenal in itself, it is also one of the most useful of herbs. It may be used as a spring tonic and potherb (heat or drying destroys the stinging components in the hairs), as a milk stimulant for breastfeeding mothers, and to enhance egg production among poultry (as a tea for the former, dried and powdered herb for the latter). It can also be useful as cattle fodder and as a healing beer, and is an old remedy for arthritis ("urtification" was flogging the affected body parts with nettle branches). It can be made into a dye, and its fibers, woven into a cloth, were said to compete with the finest linen. This Martian plant can be used, with care, for the most beneficial ends, but if incautiously mishandled, it will hurt. The stinging can be nullified by crushing any demulcent herb growing nearby. Dock is the one traditionally recommended, since it always grows near nettle.[8] But plantain or purslane will work, or anything from which you can coax a few emergency drops of soothing viscosity—whether or not you recite the traditional spell:

> *Nettle in, dock out.*
> *Dock rub nettle out!*

The 28th Path: Aries
Tiger Lily, Geranium

Crowley writes

> ... Geranium has a scarlet variety which is precisely the colour of Aries in the King Scale. The Tiger Lily is a traditional attribution.[9]

This geranium is always the scarlet one, found ubiquitously as a spring bedding plant. A tender perennial (as they call annuals nowadays), it can be over-wintered inside with care and enough light. The tiger lily, *Lilium trigrinum*, is an Asian native, cultivated there mainly for its edible roots, that has naturalized itself in North America and the U. K. Its color ranges from red-orange to scarlet, always heavily speckled with black. The pollen is poisonous, and the tuberous root can be bitter. That's it; the color and the poisonous pollen and bitter root gain its place in Aries' train.

The 24th Path: Scorpio
Cactus

In addition to cactus, Crowley also mentions nettle, in the note on the 24th path of Scorpio:

> The cactus has watery pulp and poisonous spikes. The nettle is treacherously Martial. All treacherous and poisonous plants may be attributed to Scorpio.[10]

Scorpio is the feminine of the two signs ruled by Mars. Thus, to the classical astrologer, she compounded all the negative Martian traits with the tired old antique attitudes toward the feminine, making Scorpio even worse than Aries (hard as that may be to imagine). To gain a little illumination from the point of view of the tarot, Aries is given to the Emperor card, while Scorpio belongs to the Death card. And while it is true that, in the end, Death is Emperor of all living things, it's still troubling to be reminded of that fact.

The 27th Path: Mars
Absinthe, Rue

Absinthe: I believe that by absinthe, Crowley meant absinthium, an old name for wormwood (*Artemesia absinthium*). One curiosity is that one would think all members of the genus *Artemesia* (numbering 180 or so) would belong to Artemis. Mrs. Grieve quotes Apuleius (ok, the Pseudo-Apuleius) in his *Herbarium* stating that the goddess Diana (Artemis) found them and gave the plants to the great physician, Chiron the Centaur, who developed their medicinal use and named them after her. She then quotes a section of July's *Husbandry*, by Tusser (1577), that pairs off this path's plants:

> While Wormwood hath seed get a handful or twaine
> To save against March, to make flea to refraine;
> Where chamber is sweeped and Wormwood is strowne.
> What saver is better (if physick be true)
> For places infected than Wormwood and Rue?
> It is a comfort for hart and the braine,
> And therefore to have it is not in vaine.[11]

Mrs. Grieve goes on to note that "with the exception of Rue, Wormwood is the bitterest herb known."[12] This bitterness is why these herbs correspond to the 27th path. Mars rules all bitter, biting tastes, and *Artemesia absinthum* has long been thought to belong to him. *Potter's Therapeutics* mentions anise, marjoram and angelica in the liqueur absinthe and notes that it:

> is an alcoholic solution of the oil [of Wormwood]. . . . Its continued use produces various nervous symptoms, morning nausea and vomiting, also a tendency towards eliptiform convulsions. The bitter constituent of Absinthium is stimulant to the digestive organs, but the oil is a narcotic poison. It increases the cardiac action, and produces tremor, stupor . . . involuntary evacuations, and stertorous breathing. It is but little used in medicine, only as a stomachic tonic to treat dyspepsia.[13]

Maybe my idea of a romantic 19th-century French absinthe bar with its artistic patrons is, well, misinformed.

Rue: Mrs. Grieve tells us that rue leaves emit a powerful, disagreeable odor and have an exceedingly bitter, acrid, and nauseous taste. Rue was formerly in the official pharmacopoeia, but by the publication of *Potter's Therapeutics* (the edition I'm using is the 14th, published in 1926), its use had been abandoned. This work describes rue as an active irritant, the oil applied locally producing heat, inflammation, and vesication [blistering].

Important *caveat*: approach rue in the heat of midday with discretion, because merely brushing it against bare skin can raise a rash. Such are rue's powers, earning it its place of honor in the train of Mars.

Chapter Four

The Plants of the Sun

Tiphareth: Acacia, Bay, Laurel, Vine
19th Path, Leo: Sunflower
30th Path, the Sun: Sunflower, Laurel, Heliotrope

"I married Isis on the fifth day of May . . . " —Bob Dylan

In Astrology, the Sun is the giver and sustainer of life. In the chart, it signifies the ego. On the Tree of Life, it aligns with Ruach, that part of the consciousness that, I was taught, thinks it is the self but is not. In the zodiac, the Sun rules Leo; in the body, the Sun is the heart, the circulatory system, and the back. The Sun is the ruler, in many ways: it represents the monarch of any country, the lead actor in any play, the CEO of any company, the boss of any mob. It's the center and the central actor in any concern, and all else revolves around it.[1]

The importance of the Sun and the sign it occupies is why sun-sign Astrology works more often than not. As the ego, it rules how natives relate to themselves, always colored by the sign they're in. I'm painting with broad strokes here, and do not mean to diminish the importance of the Moon and its sign—just as important to the emotional, inner self as the Sun is to the persona of the native—nor of the thousands of other points in any chart that need to be analyzed, weighed, and synthesized before a balanced and accurate interpretation can be given.

However, the Sun, and its sign, Leo, were of such significance to Crowley that he always implied Leo was his own sign, even though he was an October 12th Libra with a Leo ascendant and first-house Leo Uranus. His most public personal sigil, of course, is the one portraying either the symbol for Leo, with the Sun inserted in the top arc of the sign, or an erect phallus and testicles, seen head-on, as it were—or both, really. It's safe to say that Crowley, and every other Leo rising, really identifies with that Ascendant.

The Sun is as central to the horoscope as the heart is to the body, and as Tiphareth, the Realm of the Sun, is to the Tree of Life. It occupies the center of the Tree, and is the critical balance point between the lower, petty human self, and the higher, more cosmic self.

Ficino writes:

Now our own soul ... puts forth a general force of life everywhere within us—especially through the heart as the source of the fire which is the nearest thing to the soul. In the same way the World-soul, which is active everywhere, unfolds in every place its power of universal life principally through the Sun. Accordingly, some thinkers say the entire Soul, both in us and in the universe, dwells in any member but most of all in the heart and in the Sun.[2]

It is difficult to overstate the vital importance of the Sun to life on our planet, or the its significance in the birth chart to the life of the body and of the consciousness. Without the Sun, life on Earth would not exist. Like the green vegetation of the Earth that requires sunlight for photosynthesis, our bodies require Vitamin D—the only vitamin manufactured by the skins of animals, including us, by exposure to sunlight. Vitamin D is essential in metabolizing calcium and imperative to our physical well-being.

The Sun also signifies an area of magical operation. Lévi summarizes them as "works of light and riches," including works concerning children, creativity, fame, superiors, vitality and health of the body, love affairs, and drama or theatrics. The magical alphabet gives the magical powers of the Sun, or Tiphareth, as the Vision of the Harmony of Things, also the Mysteries of the Crucifixion.

The Plants of Tiphareth, The Sphere of the Sun
Acacia, Bay Laurel, Vine, [N.B. also Oak and Gorse]

Crowley writes of Tiphareth:

> The Oak is also, and more properly, attributed to Tiphareth because it was the sacred tree of the Druids, the representative in the vegetable kingdom of the Sun. Its strength is also taken as harmonious with that quality in man. Futhermore, the Acorn is peculiarly phallic, and this is properly to be attributed to Tiphareth because in this case the phallic symbol contains in itself the essence of the being to be reproduced. The Acacia is placed here as a symbol of resurrection as in the rituals of Free Masonry. The Bay and Laurel are sacred to Apollo, the Vine to Dionysus.[3]

Oak: Tiphareth is one of oak's several placements on the Tree. Overlapping symbolism may be confusing at first. However, neither botanical symbolism nor mythography are exact sciences—nor do I think they should be. What we're seeing with oak attributed to the 5th, 21st, and 32nd path 32 *(bis)*, as well as to the 6th sephirah, are different aspects of one plant as it pertains to the different paths on the Tree of Life. Depending on the path, the oak is considered kingly (21st path, Jupiter), warlike (5th Sephirah, hardness of wood for weapons), and stable (32nd path at the base of the Tree of Life).

Bay/Laurel: Bay and laurel are interchangeable names for the same plant, *Larus nobilis*. Even the Latin name of this plant reflects its royal, "noble" status. The reader will recall how Olympic athletes—kings among men!—and Roman emperors wore wreaths of laurel to denote their exalted status. Mrs. Grieve tells us that the leaves, berries, and oil have excitant and narcotic properties. She also recounts the old story that the Delphic oracles made use of bay leaves—a claim now discounted by the geologic examinations at Delphi. The priestesses really didn't need to chew bay leaves when they had such lovely streams of psychoactive gases to inhale. I also direct the reader to the phrase *In vino, veritas* for the Dionysian side of this equation.

As Crowley notes, bay/laurel is associated with Apollo, the primary Greek Sun god. Apollo's connection with bay/laurel stems from his lust for the nymph Daphne. As the god was just about to catch her, Daphne prayed to her river-god father, who turned her into a bay tree. To console himself, he made a wreath of laurel leaves to wear.[4]

The Vine: Vines produce the grapes that are crushed to make wine, the communion of choice for several millennia. Dionysus, Apollo's younger brother and patron god of wine, is attributed to Tiphareth as another sacrificial god. Dionysus, born Zagreus, "the horned child crowned with serpents" of Zeus and Persephone, was torn to pieces[5] and eaten by Titans at the instigation of Hera. Only his heart remained. Zeus took the heart and used it to create Semele (in other variations, he fed it to her). Zeus then impregnated Semele in the form of a shower of gold, and she conceived Dionysus. When she, foolishly as it *always* turns out, asked to see the father of her child in his true form, she was blasted by a lightning bolt. Dad once again snatched his son from death and sewed him into his own divine "thigh" to complete the gestation period. You can't keep a good god down!

Dionysus, for my money, has the most interesting history of transformations of any Olympian. Snatched up, torn to bits, and boiled up for a snack, he was reconstituted by his grandmother, Rhea, and appears as a goat, a stag, a bull, or a ram, depending on the particular point in, or version of, his biography you are referencing.[6] What's surprising is that he ever had the time to invent wine.

Since these two gods appear at Tiphareth, we could take Apollo as the "higher" or more ordered, civilized aspect of consciousness, and Dionysus as the "lower," more chaotic. While this may be true in the most superficial and arbitrary way, the relationship between these two gods is much richer than that. Nietzsche, in his *Birth of Tragedy*, has the whole of civilization produced by the tension between the twin poles of Apollo and Dionysus. That they are, at last, identified as one speaks to the meaning of Tiphareth. Apollo reigns over form; Dionysus is a force that cannot be denied—not by Hera, or Titans, or Kings, or even by the tribe of Amazons.

Acacia: The other plant attributed to Tiphareth is acacia, which, as Crowley mentions, figures prominently in the lore of Freemasonry. A branch of acacia marked the grave of the Master Hiram Abiff, who was murdered by three corrupt junior Masons building Solomon's Temple. This ensures the Master Builder's place among all sacrificed gods residing in Tiphareth.[7] The acacia is a thorny member of the locust, or pea, family. It was, writes Hageneder:

> of great importance in ancient Egypt, both practically and spiritually. Of the native trees, it was the most widespread and also the most useful. . . . The wood was strong enough to form the main timbers of the hulls and ribs of small ships. . . . Most importantly, the original sacred barge of Osiris at the temple of Thebes was made from acacia. . . . The acacia was the guardian of this promise [of immortality], because it protected Osiris' mummy while his soul embraced the universe. Inscriptions call him "the solitary one in the acacia," and inscribed images show the god as a mummy sheltered by the tree.[8]

Gorse: Crowley appends gorse to the list of plants of Tiphareth as the sacred flower of the Argentum Astrum (A∴A∴). He also includes ash (Yggdrasil, the World-Tree). "Aswata, the world-Fig, should also be attributed here as the Tree itself in the microcosm."[9]

Path 19: Leo
Sunflower

It is unclear whether, by sunflower, Crowley means the New World native *Helianthus annuus*, or the Old World *Calendula off.*, the pot marigold. I'm going to assume that, if he had meant *Calendula*, he would have listed it that way; I assume this because the *Helianthus annuus* is so very well-placed here. Mrs. Grieve gives an alternate name for it, *Corona solis*; indeed, "Crown of the Sun" describes it exactly. Its great, shaggy, golden head, if not phototropic as was once alleged, at least looks like our Sun, and also closely resembles the head and mane of the lion. (We'll find phototropism enough in the heliotrope, on the 30th path.) This plant was sacred to the Incan Sun God; the Spanish carried this vegetative gold back to Europe, where its hybridization began.

The giant sunflower, the common one, is an enormous plant, growing up to eight or nine, or even 12 feet tall.[10] A field of sunflowers in full bloom in the late summer (the time of Leo, to be sure) is a stunning sight to behold. In terms of the "medicinal" properties of the giant sunflower, the only one I can find relating to Tiphareth is that using sunflower oil in cooking raises good and lowers bad cholesterol, and is thus recommended for heart health.

The 30th Path: The Sun
Sunflower, Laurel, Heliotrope [N.B. also Galangal]

Crowley calls these attributions "obvious." The heliotropes (*Heliotropium* spp.) are sweet-smelling plants that are fully, well, heliotropic, since, as Mrs. Grieve puts it:

> . . . it follows the course of the Sun. After opening it gradually turns from the east to the west and during the night turns again to the east to meet the rising sun.[11]

Galangal: Crowley goes on to write that, in addition to the "obvious" attributions of sunflower, laurel, and heliotrope, "Galangal is specially sacred to the Sun; it is of the Ginger Family."[12] Galangal (*Alpinia officinarum*) was introduced into the pharmacopeia of Europe by the writings of the Arabic physicians Rhazes and Avicenna (Ibn Sina), and was first recorded by Ibn Khurdadbah, in 879, as a trade good from the Orient. Hildegard of Bingen found galangal to be the most effective heart remedy in her repertory:

> Whoever has heart pain and is weak in the heart should instantly eat enough galangal, and he or she will be well again.[13]

Hildegard goes on to say that "If there would be a drug to wake up the dead, then galangal would be the first choice."[14] The reader will doubtless recall that in the microcosm, the Sun rules the heart.

Chapter Five

THE PLANTS OF VENUS

Netzach: Rose
14th Path, the planet Venus: Myrtle, Rose, Clover
16th Path, Taurus: Mallow
22nd Path, Libra: Aloe.

"O Heavenly Harlot, Lover of all, refuser of none . . . "
—Lon Milo DuQuette

Venus is the complement and balance of Mars. She is the sexually active woman, that part of the psyche requiring another for completion. Only in relationship to the other is she fulfilled; once conjoined, the products of the union can emerge, whether they are of the body or of the creative spirit. Contrasting Venus with the Moon, Crowley, knowing her power, writes:

> Venus . . . the passive—the receptive. She receives, and she gives back in kind what she receives. . . . Woman! Either in the form of . . . Lilith, the demon queen . . . or Woman the goddess, who blazes in the heavens, clothed with the Sun, the Moon her footstool, and crowned with the zodiac, the planets clustered in her hands. . . . gaiety, mirth and happy companionings are of her making. The arts are her handmaidens, music is for her dancing feet, scents delight her, and touch is hers. . . . Beauty, allurement, passion, graciousness are all hers . . . [1]

In her, we find mythologized the life-force itself, relegated by the patriarchy to the flirt, mistress, lover, or harlot. By Roman times, her child, Eros—considered by Plato's Socrates to be, after Chaos, the oldest god, and "in very truth . . . the ancient source of all our highest good"—was demoted to the chubby, annoying little sprite with the arrows.

Mars, as stated, needs to be *doing* something; Venus needs to *belong*, to be with someone. Crowley's comments above emphasize her receptivity to the planets aspecting her. Adverse aspects will produce a native who is described by Morin as: "Timid, idle . . . and bothersome in love affairs. . ., imprudently and unfortunately jealous, . . . addicted to indecent desires, disreputable . . . "[2]

Well-placed, however, we find the native:

> ... charming ... merciful, peace-making, cheerful, sociable ...
> devoted to dancing, singing, music, and dining, elegant and charming
> ... playful ... fortunate ... in love affairs and friendships, kind ...
> unable to endure hard work, quarrels, anger ... and easily
> reconciled.[3]

Venus' dual nature is noted above by Crowley, as well as throughout *The Book of Thoth*. He refers his readers to the formula of copper as the emblem of her two sides. We find these again in his discussion of trump V, The Hierophant (Taurus), where he directs us to *The Book of the Law*, chapter 1, verse 57: "[T]here are love and love. There is the dove, and there is the serpent." He writes further of Taurus:

> The ruler of this sign is Venus; she is represented by the woman
> standing before the Hierophant. Chapter III of *The Book of the Law*,
> verse xi, reads:
>   "Let the woman be girt with a sword before me." This woman
> represents Venus as she now is in this new aeon; no longer the mere
> vehicle of her male counterpart, but armed and militant.[4]

This is not your languid floozie of a Venus, the dysfunctional girl characterized by "... a faded movie queen, lying back on her divan ... fat and vainglorious, eating chocolates."[5] Those elements show Aphrodite's less attractive side, coming directly from Greek mythology, flirting, cajoling, tricking, seducing, and charming any and all who come her way. However, any attempt to reduce her to a mere sex-driven bimbo is incomplete, at the very least, when some other aspects, more aligned with Crowley's vision of her in Atu V, are considered. Robert Graves notes that:

> As Goddess of Death-in Life, Aphrodite earned many titles which
> seem inconsistent with her beauty and complaisance. At Athens, she
> was called the Eldest of the Fates and sister of the Erinnyes:[6] and
> elsewhere Melaenis ("black one") ...; Scotia ("dark one");
> Androphonos ("man-slayer"); and even according to Plutarch, Epi-
> tymbria ("of the tombs").[7]

What better titles for the Woman Girt with a Sword do we need?

The Plants of Netzach: The Sphere of Venus
Rose

Crowley says that the rose has always belonged to Venus. In *The Goddess of Love*, Geoffrey Grigson writes:

> One fancy of the Greeks was that roses and Aphrodite were born simultaneously. At the moment when the young goddess took shape in the sea from the sperm of Ouranos a new shrub appeared on earth. The assembly of the blessed gods spilt drops of nectar on its scions, and each drop became a rose.[8]

By the 2nd century B.C.E., the rose belonged unquestionably to Aphrodite. Pausanius, in his *Description of Greece*, details the marketplace of Elis, mentioning the nearby sanctuary to the Graces, and the three statues there.

> One of them holds a rose, the middle one a die, and the third a small branch of myrtle . . . The reason for their holding these things may be guessed to be this. The rose and the myrtle are sacred to Aphrodite . . . while the Graces are of all deities the nearest related to Aphrodite. As for the die, it is the plaything of youths and maidens, who have nothing of the ugliness of old age.[9] On the right of the Graces is an image of Love, standing on the same pedestal.[10]

Most people do love the rose, even without the fragrance, which has been bred out of florists' roses, sacrificed on the altar of commerce to produce a large and long-lasting bloom for their trade. The cultivation of the rose is ancient. Roses are found in the frescoes of Minoan homes, *c.* 1500 B.C.E., as well as in Egyptian tomb paintings of the same period.

Culpeper, as writers before him, assigned the damask rose to Venus. This was the rose most popular in the Roman Empire—with its intense and intoxicating fragrance, semi-double to double blooms, in colors from white and white touched with red, to pink and the red so beloved of roses today. It was the fact of the rose's wild popularity in Rome, particularly Nero's attachment to it, that led the early Church to despise it as a "symbol of depravity." However, by the early 15th century, the goddess had regained her ecclesiastical imprimatur through the association of the (white) rose with the Blessed Virgin.

Generally, whenever you have a discussion of roses in antique times, the variety under discussion is the apothecary rose, *Rosa gallica officinalis.* Rose oil was not distilled until late, and essential oil of roses was not known to the ancients; they compounded the petals with "carrier" materials to hold the fragrance. Avicenna is credited with the first preparation of rose water in the tenth century. The famous attar (otto) of roses was discovered by pure serendipity sometime *circa* the late 16th century, at the nuptials of a royal Persian couple. Rosewater filled the canals upon which the royal wedding-barge was to float and, when that canal water steeped in Persia's blistering sun, the essential rose oil separated and floated to the surface.

> It was skimmed off and found to be an exquisite perfume ... [Immediately] ... manufacture of Otto of Roses was commenced in Persia ... [11]

Today, the primary medical use of the rose is in aromatherapy. Essential oil of rose is used to address depression, insomnia, women's complaints, and cosmetic issues. However, as far as I'm concerned, were the rose only to provide beauty to eyes and olfactories, she has quite justified her existence. Daphne Filiberti writes of David Austin's famous remark, "Fragrance is the other half of the beauty of a rose":

> Austin has said that scent is the *soul of the rose*. It is something that we can not hold in our hands, [something] which is always shifting and changing.[12]

This statement echoes precisely Dion Fortune's comments on Netzach in *The Mystical Qabbalah*:

> In Netzach force is still relatively free-moving, being bound only into exceedingly fluidic and ever-shifting shapes ... flowing backwards and forwards over the boundaries of manifestation in an exceedingly elusive manner.[13]

14th Path: Venus
Myrtle, Rose, Clover

Myrtle: Ovid, in his *Fasti*, tells us the myrtle belongs to Aphrodite because, when Venus-Aphrodite came ashore and was wringing the water from her hair, she saw that she was being watched by a coarse crowd of satyrs—

And so hid her bodily parts with myrtle
And was safe.[14]

Malcolm Stuart, editor of the inestimable *Encyclopedia of Herbs and Herbalism,* remarks of *Myrtus communi:*

> [It] was almost certainly because the aromatic leaves bear a resemblance to the females' pudenda that Myrtle has been dedicated to Venus, that it has been considered an aphrodisiac, and carried by Israeli brides, for example, at their weddings.[15]

The leaves of the plant are indeed almond-shaped,[16] with a central vein separating the two halves of the leaf that gently plump out as they separate, and do thereby evoke such an image. Barbara Walker, in her remarkable *Women's Dictionary of Symbols and Sacred Objects,* goes a bit further than mere "resemblance"; she maintains that the "Greek word for myrtle meant also female genitals. The myrtle berry (*to myrton*) meant the clitoris."[17]

As a symbol of divine generosity, myrtle is among the plants Adam was given on his expulsion from Eden: "wheat, chief of foods; the date, chief of fruits; and the myrtle, chief of scented flowers," as the Moldenkes put it in their *Plants of the Bible.*[18] J. C. Cooper relates that the myrtle has been used throughout Eastern and Western cultures as a plant symbolizing joy, peace, success, initiation, baptism, success in marriage, fame, and gentiles converted to Christianity. Professor Cooper agrees with Robert Graves that "Myrtle is a vital essence and transmits the breath of life, and is symbolic of life germinating and rebirth and life renewed."[19]

The myrtle was sacred to Aphrodite in all her aspects. Pausanius mentions "an image of Aphrodite in Temnus made of a living myrtle-tree."[20] Grigson remarks that "[for] the Greeks, in a frank way, these scented leaves and scented stems and scented flowers indicated love, and its pleasures. . . . brides wore myrtle for what was to come on the wedding night . . . [and] not as a modern white wedding symbol of innocence and virginity."[21]

Robert Graves looks at the matter from his customary extra-dimensional abode:

> [The] myrtle was sacred to the Love-goddess Aphrodite all over the Mediterranean, partly because it grows best near the sea shore, partly because of its fragrance; nevertheless, it was the tree of death. Myrto,

or Myrtea, or Myrtoessa was a title of hers and the pictures of her sitting with Adonis in the myrtle-shade were deliberately misunderstood by the Classical poets. She was not vulgarly courting him, as they pretended, but was promising him Life-in-death; for myrtle was a token of the resurrection of the dead King of the year.[22]

I'll only mention here the Rose Cross of Tiphareth.

Clover: Although Crowley lists clover as one of the "traditional" plants of this path, I haven't had much luck turning up this association. Be that as it may, 777's magical alphabet does not specify which of the clovers it means, so use any of them in ritual work—either the white sweet clover (*Melitotus alba*), yellow sweet clover (*Melitotus officianalis*), or red clover (*Trifolium pretense*). I'd use either of the *Melitotus* species, the "*officianalis*" clover of the Materia Medica, or the other—both of them are named "sweet" (*mel* is the root of the word "honey") and thus belong to Venus. Even red clover is used for female reproductive-system support, and is thus under her reign, so you'd be safe using it as well. In my opinion, it is the sense of "being in clover"—that is, to be in favorable circumstances—that lands it on Venus' list.

16th Path: Taurus
Mallow

Crowley again refers to mallow's listing here as traditional. The members of this family that I've grown (hollyhock and okra, notably) will keep growing up. And up. And up.

This Eurasian native is a member of the *Malvaceae* family, which includes the hollyhocks, the hibiscus, and some thousand other plants. The magical alphabet's mallow is most likely *Malva sylvestris* (*sylvestris* means "of the woods" and refers always to the wild plant). "Mallow," from the Latin *malva*, means soft—like Venus—and refers to the demulcent (soothing, softening) action of the plant. Mrs. Grieve writes of a species of mallow that was discovered at the time of her writing: "[All] of which not only contain much mucilage, but are totally devoid of unwholesome properties."[23]

Leave it to Venus to rule a huge garden family, not one member of which has any adverse property whatsoever. The common mallow was a very popular remedy among ancient herbalists for many complaints. Pliny mentions that its seeds sprinkled upon the genitals promote lust, as will tying three mallow roots on the body near the area in question.

It is an herb of Venus, after all. Culpeper attributes the plant to Venus, and suggests that the "smaller kind of Mallow, with white flowers" (the "low mallow," *M. rotundifolia*, which has the same properties as *M. sylvestris*) has a more pleasant taste.

The common mallow is easy to grow and looks like a half-pint version of its close relative, the hollyhock. It is, likewise, a biennial or short-lived perennial. The most readily available cultivar is *Malva sylvestris*, 'Zebrina,' which blooms a lovely striped mauve or soft purple on flowers perhaps two inches across on an upright stem three feet or so tall. I had Zebrina for several years, self-sowing in one of my borders. I grew it in front of the black hollyhock, making a striking contrast.

22nd Path: Libra
Aloe

Aloe vera is a thick-leaved succulent native to Southern and Eastern Africa, but naturalized throughout the tropical world and well-known by ancient herbalists. Pliny records twenty-nine remedies using the plant, and reports it as the best purgative known.[24] He also mentions its excellent use for healing wounds of all sorts, and indeed, aloe remains a popular herb for either of these uses. The ancient Egyptians knew and used aloe as well, and the plant is mentioned in the Bible several times. However, the Old Testament "aloe" was almost assuredly *Aquilaria agallocha*, the eaglewood tree, or, more commonly, lignum-aloes.

The juice of the aloe vera, applied immediately to burns, will instantly provide relief and speed healing. A pot of aloe, grown in a gritty soil (you can buy bags of "cactus" soil at your local nursery) and placed in a sunny kitchen window will, I assure you, come in very handy. Keep some frozen leaves in a well-sealed baggie and apply directly to burns or any other skin irritation. However, unless you are gardening in a tropical zone, don't attempt to grow aloe outside, as it is a very tender perennial.

I'd also like to point out that the juice of both the aloe and the mallow are mucilaginous and slimy, and remind me of nothing as much as a woman's sexual secretions. Perfect for these two plants of Venus!

Chapter Six

THE PLANTS OF MERCURY

Hod: Moly, Anhalonium Lewinii
12th Path, Mercury: Vervain, Herb Mercury, Marjoram, Palm
17th Path, Gemini: Hybrids, Orchids
20th Path, Virgo: Snowdrop, Lily, Narcissus

"Sometimes I don't think about nothin' but the Monkey Man."
—the Traveling Wilburys

Although Mercury is important astrologically, he does not have the "weight" that he does in the magical spheres. Transiting Mercury moves so quickly that his effect in our daily lives is fleeting, unnoticed until he turns retrograde (and thereby provides sufficient reason for any screw-up whatsoever). In magick—is there anything Mercury does not touch? When I was taught beginning Qabala, back when the rocks were still warm to the touch, my teacher impressed upon us that the workings of ritual magick were found in the sphere of Hod. Certainly, tradition holds that Mercury, in his role as Thoth, the Thrice-Great Hermes, was the original conveyor of the arts magical.

One can easily see this tension between the trivial and the profound in the two sections on Mercury in *The General Principles of Astrology*. The first shows little any astrologer wouldn't already know, confirming that Crowley's Astrology is, at heart, very traditional. Here, we read the standard Mercury fare—"cold, dry, earthy," "lucky or unlucky" depending on other planetary relationships; Mercury the Trickster; well-disposed, giving an active strong intellect; poorly disposed, an ill wind indeed, giving an unprincipled, shiftless mind.

This sort of thing can be found in any Astrology text. However, let's look at the next section, "Mercury Symbolically Considered":

Hermes ... is the ... vital intelligence of God ... the wisdom of the Creator, the Logos or Word by whom all things came into being.... [Swifter] than the lightning, for he is thought itself, wherein the lightning lives. The divine consciousness is free from time and space ... and so Hermes, being the thought of Deity, transcends such bounds.... He is the master also of magick, and the patron of all those who seek after God by solitude and meditation.[1]

Mythologically, the Greek Hermes was a difficult god in ways hard to imagine—unless you remember that his metal is quicksilver, the living silver, the metal that moves. It is as easy to corral quicksilver as to contain Hermes. Soon after his birth, Hermes rustled Apollo's sacred cattle herd, invented the first sacrificial rites, invented the lyre, and then traded it to Apollo for the cattle he had stolen. He so impressed his father, Zeus, and the other gods with those sacrifices that nobody even noticed he had finessed for himself a place on Mount Olympus. He got himself appointed as Zeus' official herald, and was thus awarded the broad-brimmed traveler's hat, the ribbon-bedecked herald's staff (the *caduceus*[2]), and the winged sandals that became his emblems. He invented fire and the making of it, gambling, divination with knuckle-bones, the alphabet, astronomy, the musical scale, boxing and gymnastics, weights and measures, the cultivation of the olive-tree, and, oh yes, became Psychopompos.

This is a remarkable catalogue for any god, but Hermes is not just any god.[3]

Mercury is the most dual-natured of the planets. He speaks truth and lies. He represents the most sublime leaps of intuition into the very mind of God, but he also rules gossip and gadding aimlessly about. He cheated his way onto Olympus, but only after he had invented the rites of worship. With this planet, we're introduced to verbal deftness, artistic creativity, thievery, travel, commerce, realms charted and unknown, magick, and the passing from life into death. Mercury is outside the categories of good and evil. When we travel with Hermes, we pass beyond stifling consensual morality and move directly into the Will.

Another side of Hermes is indicated in his title as "Lord of the Roads," referring to the piles of stones called "herms," sometimes robustly ithyphallic. These ancient altars to Hermes marked the boundaries of roads, regions, and countries.

In *The Book of Thoth*, Crowley described Mercury as the embodiment of the Word, representing

> ... both truth and falsehood, wisdom and folly. Being the unexpected, he unsettles any established idea, and therefore appears tricky. He has no conscience, being creative ... He cannot be understood, because he is the Unconscious Will.[4]

Therefore, one can consider that Hermes delineates both our psychological and physical roads, borders, and boundaries. Pretty impressive, for a little ball of a planet not 30° from the Sun.

The Plants of Hod: The Sphere of Mercury
Moly, Anhalonium Lewinii

Moly: The attribution of moly to Mercury raises the fact that the plant's identity is one of the most controversial questions relating to any plants mentioned in ancient writings. Crowley comments that moly:

> is mentioned in Homer as having been given by Hermes to Ulysses to counteract the spells of Circe. It has a black root and white blossoms, which again suggests the dual currents of energy.[5]

Linnaeus first classified this plant as the *Allium magicum*, the magic onion, giving the nod to its Homeric reputation. Theophrastus suggested that Homer's moly was the *Epimedean Squill*. Pliny notes, in *The Natural History*, that the moly is yellow-flowered, and not, as Homer maintains, white. Many authors suggest that Homer's moly was a strictly mythological—i.e., imaginary—plant.

Moly—*Allium moly*, now often referenced as *A. moly luteum*—is an onion. At some point during Elizabethan times, all ornamental onions became known as "mollies." Hermes chose this powerful herb, with its ability to counteract all bewitchments and poisons, to give to Ulysses. As Crowley notes above (as described by Homer, anyway), it has the black-and-white coloring suggestive of the twin nature of the god. Another point to remember about the onion is that each bulb consists of many layers. It is all too easy, when removing the layers to get to the "real" plant, to end up with piles of layers and a big handful of nothing. Perhaps a key to the connection between moly and Hermes lies in the layering of the leaves rather than in the composition of the layers.

Anhalonium lewenii: The peyote cactus, *Anhalonium lewenii*, is one of a number of New World cacti with hallucinogenic properties. The Nahuatl word for it is *peyotl*. Several members of this cactus family produce mescal buttons, which are the tops of the plant, cut and dried. All contain basically the same psychoactive constituents. The main one is mescaline, weaker than, but similar to, LSD. Mescal's scarcity lies in the fact that so very little of the plant grows above the surface of the ground—at most four inches. It is native to the limestone deserts of Mexico and southern Texas. The Peyote cult, which uses the plant in its rituals, is at least 2000 to 3000 years old.

The Spanish quickly came to condemn peyote for its "satanic trickery" and brutally persecuted the adherents of the cult. The Native peoples have fought for centuries for the peyote ceremony to be accepted along with every other legitimate religious ritual. They finally succeeded with the official acceptance of the Native American Church, in which the communion service consists of a night-long ritual following the ingestion of mescal buttons.

Although it has been used for untold generations by other cultures, peyote's place in Western psychopharmacology is more recent. By 1954, when Aldous Huxley wrote *The Doors of Perception*, the use of mescaline in psychiatric pharmacology was well-established. Huxley notes that psychologists experimenting with it concurred in assigning to mescaline a position among drugs of unique distinction. Administered in suitable doses, it changes the quality of consciousness more profoundly, and yet is less toxic, than any similar substance. In his own mescaline experience, Huxley was accompanied by a colleague who taped the occasion and questioned the author during his trip so there would be an accurate record of the adventure. Huxley writes of understanding:

> *Istigkeit*—wasn't that the word Meister Eckhart liked to use? "Is-ness." . . .
>
> I continued to look at the flowers, and in their living light I seemed to detect the qualitative equivalent of breathing. . . . My eyes traveled from the rose to the carnation, and from that feathery incandescence to the smooth scrolls of sentient amethyst which were the iris. The Beatific Vision, *Sat Chit Ananda*, Being-Awareness-Bliss—for the first time I understood, not on the verbal level . . . but precisely and completely what those prodigious syllables referred to.[6]

Huxley later describes his immediate and total apprehension of every Zen *koan* he'd encountered, as well as the deepest levels of meaning in Marx Brothers' movies. In other words, the standard psychedelic itinerary. Lord Hermes led Huxley across the border, from the state of consensual reality into the inner realms of Being itself. Crowley wrote that peyote has "as one of its principal characteristics the power to produce very varied and brilliant colour visions."[7]

Dion Fortune might have been tripping with Aldous (only kidding!) when she wrote thus of Hod in *The Mystical Qabalah*:

The Spiritual Experience assigned to this Sephirah is the Vision of Splendour, which is the realisation of the glory of God manifesting in the created world. The initiate of Hod sees behind the appearance of created things and discerns their Creator, and in the realization of the splendour of Nature as the garment of the Ineffable he received his illumination . . . [8]

The 12th Path: Mercury
Vervain, Herb Mercury, Marjoram, Palm

Vervain: *Verbena officinalis* is also called the herb of grace, holy plant (*Hiera botane*), divine weed, and *Herba sacra*. It was used so much in ancient Roman rituals as a cleansing plant that the name *Verbena* came to mean "altar plant." It was regarded as so critical to Roman spiritual life that it had its own annual festival, the *Verbenalia*. Pliny recounts that the Romans were introduced to vervain by the Celts. His accompanying rant against magick is pregnant with clues on the magical properties of vervain:

> The people in the Gallic provinces make use of them both for sooth-saying purposes . . . but it is the magicians more particularly that give utterance to such ridiculous follies in reference to this plant. Persons, they tell us, if they rub themselves with it will be sure to gain the object of their desires. . . . they say, too, that it must be gathered about the rising of the Dog-star—but so as not to be shone upon by sun or moon—and that honey-combs and honey must be first presented to the earth by way of expiation. They tell us also that a circle must first be traced around it with iron; after which it must be taken up with the left hand, and raised aloft.[9]

As you may imagine, Vervain was, and is, one of the most indispensable items in the magical herb cupboard. It is used both in working magical spells and to protect against them. The old rhyme runs "Trefoil, vervain, St. Johnswort, and dill / Hinder witches of their will."

Mercury's ownership of vervain is not found in the earliest magical herbals. In *The Three Books on Occult Philosophy*, Agrippa assigns it to the Sun. One Qabalistic clue to Mercury's ownership of the plant is found in the Yetziratic text assigned to Hod:

> The Eighth Path is called the Absolute or Perfect Intelligence because it is the mean of the Primordial, which has no root by which it can

cleave or rest, *save in the hidden places of Gedulah, from which emanates its proper essence.*[10]

Bundles of vervain were essential in the festivals of Jupiter to sweep and purify his altars. Jupiter is the mundane chakra (i.e., the planet) of Gedulah/Chesed. Therein lies another key to vervain's Mercurial identity.

Herb Mercury: *Mercurialia annua* is also known as *Chenopodium Bonus-henricus*, "Good King Henry," and as English Mercury. It has also been called "Dog's Mercury" or "False Mercury" (*Mercurialis perennis*, a toxic plant), as well as "Children's Mercury" or "French Mercury." Oh wait, we're back to *Mercurialis annua!* From the very outset, we find ourselves in the realm of the Trickster, learning his first magical lesson: a moving target is hard to hit.

Marjoram: *Origanum marjorana*, called sweet or knotted marjoram, leads us further down the garden path of Mercury, the wily, shifty, many-turning god. The species name of this plant is *Origanum*— which means "Joy of the Mountain." In an article for *The Herbarist*, the publication of the Herb Society of America, Helen Hoyes Webster notes that, ". . . variations of this species are many. Herb gardeners are puzzled, and the nurserymen admit the nomenclatorial confusion . . . "[11]

To complicate matters, many mild types of oregano are sold as marjoram. Culpeper writes that oregano is "called also Origane, Origanum, Eastward Marjoram, Wild Marjoram, and Grove Marjoram." He ducks the whole issue of the confusion of names for this plant when he says of sweet marjoram (*Origanum Marjorana*) that it, ". . . is so well known that it is needless to write any description of it, or of either Winter Sweet Marjoram (*Origanum Heracleoticum*) or Pot Marjoram (*Origanum Onites*)."[12]

If the Mercuries in the preceding section were difficult, the marjorams/oreganos are nigh on impossible to sort out. Mrs. Grieve relates a fact that may connect marjoram mytho-historically with Hermes. "Among the Greeks, if Marjoram grew on a grave, it augured the happiness of the departed."[13] I remind the reader of Hermes' function as Psychopompos, Guide of Souls. However, in the old herbals, it is only in Culpeper that I can find anything connecting Mercury with the oreganos. I mean, marjorams.[14]

In matters of practical magick, since the various varieties of majoram are so close as to be virtually indistinguishable, feel free to follow my teacher's advice. If your oregano is of a mild sort, use it in your working. As with many other members of the Mercurialis clan, whatever you use, you'll probably hear an ethereal snickering. That's Mercury having a giggle at creating so much confusion.

Palm: Crowley writes: "The Palm is Mercurial, as being hermaphrodite."[15] J. C. Cooper writes, in *An Illustrated Encyclopedia of Traditional Symbols,* that it was also considered a self-created androgyne, and "as phallic it signifies virility and fertility, but if depicted with dates it is feminine."[16] Besides the dual-sexed qualities assigned to the palm, another Mercurial motif is that of death, and life-in-death, referring us again to Hermes Psychopompos. Ancient Egyptians laid palm fronds on mummies and in coffins. Similarly, for the early Roman Christians, the palm signified victory over death. Finally, from about 1000 B.C.E., the Tree of Life in Assyrian art increasingly resembled the shape of a date palm. All of these life/death ideas may be traced back to the Greek word for the date palm, *Phoenix dactylifera.* It was so named because the phoenix is born, ultimately dies, and is born again in the top of this tree. The phoenix was a sacred bird of Apollo. Crowley agreed with Marsilio Ficino that "Mercury is always full of Apollo."[17]

17th Path: Gemini
Hybrids, Orchids

Hybrids: These plants are the result of crossing two different cultivars of the same species. The outcome of this cross is a plant or creature that has some of the characteristics of each parent, but which itself is sterile. To ensure that you have the same plant as last season, you must plant the same hybrid seeds bought from a seed company. The old farmers saved the vegetables with the most desirable characteristics for seeds, which, because they were "open pollinated" (i.e., not hybrids), would breed true. Humankind has been "selectively breeding" for millennia—this is how the modern corn plant came into being. You'll see by this discussion that hybrid seeds, along with the booming business they foster, are securely a member of Mercury's tribe (as his title "Hermes of the Marketplace" reveals).

Orchids: We discussed the orchis (orchid) root back under the 26th path, Capricorn, and indeed Crowley refers us to that path "for obvious reasons."[18] Clearly, he means the androgynous nature of the Lord of Initiation depicted in the Devil card of Capricorn. The orchid is similarly attributable to Gemini, because its flowers are as bisexual as Mercury himself.

Of the orchid's two roots, Pliny reports:

> The larger of these tuberosities, or, as some say, the harder of the two, taken in water, is provocative of lust; while the smaller, or, in other words, the softer one, taken in goat's milk, acts as an anaphrodisiac.[19]

One can argue that one distinct qualification for the orchid's belonging to Mercury is its general adaptability. In some species, it can live entirely in the air, from which it is able to draw its nutrition (cf. Crowley's note on the 28th path [i.e., 15th path. See editor's note p. 10]).

The 20th Path: Virgo
Snowdrop, Lily, Narcissus

Crowley says of the 20th path: "The Snowdrop and Lily suggest the modest purity of the sign. Narcissus refers to the solitary tradition ... "[20]

Snowdrop: Virgo is the virgin and the zodiacal referent of the tarot card, The Hermit. Each of these plants can, by the weight of myth and tradition, be classed as goddess (virgin) plants: the snowdrop is associated with both the Christian celebration of Candlemas and the Brigid Sabbat of the pagans. The snowdrop's generic name is *Galanthus*, which means milkflower. The goddess Brigid became, in Christian times, the wet-nurse of the baby Jesus. After all, a girl's gotta work!

Further concerning the snowdrop, Malcolm Stuart writes, in *The Encyclopedia of Herbs and Herbalism*, that "recent research in Europe suggests that the plant may possess the ability to stimulate the regeneration of some nerve cells."[21] This reminds us that, anatomically, the planet Mercury rules the nervous system.

Lily: Lilies, in particular the white "Madonna" or "Easter" lilies, have such dense associations with purity that one only has to turn to any medieval or Renaissance portrayal of the Annunciation of the Blessed Virgin Mary to find them. However, in pre-Christian times, the lily belonged to Hera. Discovering that she had been tricked into suckling the infant Heracles, one of her husband's numerous by-blows, she tore the infant from her breast, flinging milk everywhere. Most of it formed the Milky Way, but some of it fell to Earth and became the lily.

Pliny mentions that lily roots boiled in wine are good for corns. This is indeed one of the main uses to which the Romans put the plant. As Mercury is the god who rules travel, obviously he appreciates healthy feet!

Narcissus: Narcissus was punished for spurning the nymph Echo. Either Aphrodite or Nemesis (according to Ovid) filled his heart with an unrequited love for himself. Unable to tear himself away from his reflection in a pool, he died of starvation, a victim of a vastly inappropriate sense of self-esteem. Goddess connections aside, and the solitary nature of Narcissus' predicament, it's difficult to find many other connections between this plant and Mercury/Hermes or Virgo/ The Hermit.

Chapter Seven

THE PLANTS OF THE MOON

Yesod: [Banyan], Mandrake, Damiana
13th Path, The Moon: Almond, Mugwort,
Hazel (as ☽), Moonwort, Ranunculus
18th Path, Cancer: Lotus

*"Diana moves with strength and will/ to bend the arrow's bow
Sending it true into the heart/ Of all I see and do"* —Ruth Barrett

The Moon in Astrology exhibits a:

> ... curiously double quality ... for its vibrations can either produce
> extreme purity and devotion to higher things, or it can make one a
> slave to the emotions.... [strongly Lunar types] are extremely sensi-
> tive and naturally absorb all kinds of influence, so they must try to
> discriminate between the true light and the false ... [1]

One approach to understanding the two sides of Luna is through
the tarot. The High Priestess card is the one associated with the Moon.
On the Tree of Life, it sits on the 13th path, which crosses the Abyss
and joins Kether (The Crown) to Tiphareth (Beauty). Beyond the
Abyss, there is no longer any physical form, for at this point, the adept
has, like "Enoch walked with God; and he was not, for God took
him."[2] In *The Book of Thoth*, Crowley describes the High Priestess as
representing:

> the most spiritual form of Isis the Eternal Virgin; the Artemis of the
> Greeks. She is clothed only in the luminous veil of light. It is impor-
> tant ... to regard Light not as the perfect manifestation of ... Spirit,
> but rather as the veil which hides that Spirit.... Thus she is light and
> the soul of light.... [and] the idea behind all form.[3]

The other end of the lunar spectrum is represented by the tarot
card, The Moon, which is associated with Pisces. The influences of this
card concur exactly with the description of the "Mother of Illusion"
referenced above. This Moon, Crowley writes, (with all due respect,
I'm sure) is:

her lowest avatar ... [She] is the waning moon, the moon of witch-craft and abominable deeds. She is the poisoned darkness which is the condition of the rebirth of the light.[4]

It is certainly outside the scope of the present work to examine the lunar goddess in any but the most cursory fashion. However, her devo-tees have long noted the various ways of experiencing her. Historical texts suggest that the original goddess of the Moon contained both the light and dark aspects in one diety.

Dion Fortune comments upon this tension:

> The study of the symbolism of Yesod reveals two apparently in-congruous sets of symbols. Upon the one hand we have the concep-tion of Yesod as the foundation of the universe, established in strength.... But upon the other hand we have the Moon symbolism, which is very fluidic, in a continual state of flux and reflux ...[5]

Crowley, of course, resolves this dilemma with his axiom "Change is Stability."

The Plants of Yesod, the Sphere of the Moon
[Banyan], Mandrake, Damiana

Banyan: Crowley brackets banyan (*Ficus benghalensis*), pointing us to its place in Kether's list, and referring us back to his note there, where we read that:

> [The] branches of the Banyan tree take fresh roots where they touch the ground and start new main stems.... It is, so to speak, the foun-dation of a system of trees as Yesod is the foundation of the branches of the Tree of Life.[6]

The tree itself is of the fig genus and exists in two species, *Ficus benghalensis* and *Ficus religiosa*. The latter is also known as the bo tree or peepul.

The bo or peepul tree is, of course, the tree under which Sidd-hartha sat until he emerged as the Enlightened One, Buddha. This plant is listed under the second sephirah, Chokhmah,[7] the realm asso-ciated with the spiritual experience of The Vision of God Face to Face. This certainly encompasses—I can only imagine—the Buddha's expe-rience under his tree.

The bo tree is considered female. The banyan, the other species of this genus, is thought of as male. This "male" aspect of the banyan tree parallels Yesod's position at the genitals on the macrocosmic man, and its magical image as "a beautiful naked man, very strong." The bo tree is named "the wish-fulfilling tree" and, due to its seeming endless expansion, represents eternal life in the Hindu system.

Mandrake: If you want one plant that exemplifies "witchcraft," mandrake (*Mandragora officianarum*) is your "booga-booga!" plant *nonpareil*. Since Pharaonic times, the mandrake has been put to such diverse uses as an antibiotic, an analgesic, a soporific, a stomachic, and, as Theophrastus writes, "a love potion."[8]

Dr. Malcolm Stuart, however, looks at the mandrake/dark magick connection differently, and suggests cold commerce alone (think of today's patented medications) are the reason for its spooky reputation:

> It was protected by the early Greek collectors who invested the root with such fictitious harmful attributes as the ability to kill a man who pulled it out of the ground.[9]

Theophrastus records some of these "magical" and "orgiastic" rites in the harvesting of mandrake:

> Thus it is said that one should draw three circles round mandrake with a sword, and cut it with one's face towards the west; and at the cutting of the second piece one should dance round the plant and say as many things as possible about the mysteries of love ...[10]

Pliny reproduces Theophrastus' comments, stressing that the very odor of the plant can render one dumb.

Flavius Josephus, dissatisfied with the existent ooky-spook content, added more, including the famous canine references. The mandrake, he writes, has a color:

> ... like to that of flame, and towards the evenings it sends out a certain ray like lightning. It is not easily taken ... but recedes from their hands, nor will yield itself to be taken quietly, until either the urine of a woman, or her menstrual blood, be poured upon it; nay, even then it is certain death to those that touch it.... It may ... be taken ... without danger ... [by digging] a trench quite round about it, till [it is almost uncovered]. They then tie a dog to it, and when the dog

tries hard to follow . . . this root is easily plucked up, but the dog dies immediately . . . [11]

The plant's ability to "send out a certain ray like lightning" toward evening may actually have a scientific basis. Under ideal weather conditions, chemicals in night's dew combine with those on the fruit's skin to produce a phosphorescence. This glow could only have contributed to the plant's eerie reputation.

Thought to have grown originally in the red earth of Paradise, Mandrake was eagerly sought by alchemists "precisely because it contained some of this unique kind of earth, which was so necessary as a catalyst in the production of the Philosopher's Stone."[12]

Mandrake seeds are notoriously hard to germinate. I will spare you my 30-year crusade and recommend that you buy some plants;[13] what you'll probably find are M. *autumnalis*, the autumn-flowering form, which has all the chemical constituents of its more famous relative. Richters Herbs sells the plants only occasionally, but usually has seeds, and claims them to sprout readily if their needs are fulfilled.[14] Once you *do* get plants, put them where they will not be disturbed, in deep, rich, rock-free soil and dappled shade.

Damiana: *Turnera diffusa*, finds itself as one of Yesod's plants because, as mentioned, Yesod in the microcosm rules the genitals. Crowley comments that "Damiana is reputed a powerful aphrodisiac, and so are Ginseng and Yohimba."[15] Damiana is a New World native. The Mayan Indians use it for lung complaints, but also more famously for its venereal effects. Like yohimbe, the herb reputedly increases blood-flow to the region of the sexual organs. Although the use of this herb is alleged to be ancient, recent scholarship in the history of Central American folk herbalism—notably Ethan Russo's *Handbook of Psychotropic Herbs*—has demonstrated that the "oldest documents cited were actually all of modern vintage."[16] Damiana as a therapeutic for sexual stimulation was debunked as early as 1906. However, damiana is still thought to be a type of herbal Viagra.

13th Path, The Moon
Almond, Mugwort, Hazel (as ☽), Moonwort, Ranunculus

Almond: Traditionally, the "almond in flower" (*Prunus amygdalus*) is the plant of Kether. This ancient native of central Asia has been an important food plant since prehistoric times. Mrs. Grieve notes that its Hebrew name, *shakad*, is very expressive: it signifies "hasty awakening" or "to watch for," hence, "to make haste." She relates this to the tree's early flowering. Aaron's Rod, one of twelve given by Moses in Numbers 17:6–8, was one such that burst into early bloom and even yielded almonds "on the morrow."

Crowley mentions the pomegranate in an aside on the plants of Yesod ("a symbol with reference to menstruation"[17]). However, in Phrygian mythology, the almond and the pomegranate are very closely related:

> In their creation myths, Agditis, a hermaphrodite monster, appeared and terrified the gods. They castrated it and turned it into the Great Mother, Cybele, causing the original unity of male and female to become divided. But from its spilled blood rose two trees, an almond and a pomegranate. Many cycles later, Attis, the divine child of the goddess Cybele, was magically conceived by the daughter of a river spirit as she ate an almond or pomegranate seed.[18]

The oldest story is that Cybele was androgynous, and where her severed male genitals touched the ground an almond tree arose, whose fruits gave birth to Attis by the daughter of the river Sangarius.

Mugwort: By the name of their genus, *Artemisia vulgaris*, you can tell that this group of plants, commonly known as mugwort, belongs to Artemis, the Lady of the Moon.[19] All the artemisias are silver or grey, or have a silvery aspect to them. In the case of mugwort, the top side of the leaf is grey-green, but the bottom shines sterling, evocative of gleaming moonlight. The "mug" is probably a reference to the ale mug, since the herb was used in brewing before the introduction of hops to impart the desired bitterness.

Culpeper, and Gerard before him, mention mugwort in the context of women's reproductive health.

Belonging to Yesod, whose spiritual experience is *A Vision of the Machinery of the Universe*, mugwort is recommended as a tea before sleep to secure prophetic dreams. You may want to cut it with chamomile and sweeten it with plenty of honey; all the artemesias are bitter to some degree, though mugwort is only mildly so.

Hazel: Crowley comments thus on *Corylus avellana*: "The Hazel is suitable for the wand of the Black magician whose typical deity is the Moon just as that of the White magician is the Sun."[20] On the other hand, he described almond as "the proper wood for the Wand of the White magician ... "[21]

Lon Milo DuQuette devotes an entire chapter in his superb *My Life With the Spirits* to its construction, and notes that:

> The three Paths of the middle pillar of the Tree of Life are GIMEL (ג), SAMEKH (ס), and TAU (ת). These three letters enumerate to 463.... The Hebrew words for "a rod of almond" ... also enumerate to the prime 463, making the almond rod the ultimate wand of power.[22]

I would, however, like to investigate the hazel just a little more deeply. I realize that Crowley was working from the "traditional" list of correspondences he received as a student in the Golden Dawn,[23] but here he seems to display an antipathy for poor old hazel that the tree simply does not warrant. After all, "hazel" in Hebrew is Heh (5), Aleph (1), Zain (7), Lamed (30), which adds up to 43 by my reckoning, *listed in 777 as equal to almond* and also described with the terms "Great" and "To rejoice." Not, in other words, anything of which to be ashamed.

Robert Graves has, as you may imagine, rather a lot to say about hazel in *The White Goddess*. He writes that the hero Fionn:

> ... was instructed by a Druid of the same name as himself to cook for him salmon fished from a deep pool of the River Boyne, and forbidden to taste it; but as Fionn was turning the fish over in the pan he burned his thumb, which he put into his mouth and so received the gift of inspiration.[24] For the salmon was a salmon of knowledge, that had fed on nuts fallen from the nine hazels of poetic art.[25]

"Hazel" in Gaelic is *Coll* and is the ninth (!) tree in the Celtic *Beth-Luis-Nion* tree alphabet. Graves continues that

> The nut in Celtic legend is always an emblem of concentrated wisdom: something sweet, compact and sustaining enclosed in a small hard shell.... [26]

I apologize for having taken such a long way around to get to my point, but finally, here it is. At the heart of this almond-hazel tension is the old, old struggle between the Great Mother, with her oracular tree, the hazel, and the invading sky-god-worshipping Indo-Europeans, who later came to comprise the Semitic tribes of the Middle East, with their rival Tree of Power, the almond. I find it suggestive that early translators of the Bible routinely substituted "hazel" for "almond." That we find both almond and pomegranate given to the 13th path, the Moon, with an attribution to "tradition" in the first place and "menstruation" in the second, gives both plants short shrift. The relationship among these plants, paths, and god/goddesses deserves a much closer scrutiny.

Moonwort: *Botrychium lunaria* is also known as *Osmunda Lunaria.* This plant is the moonwort listed in the plants of the 13th path. It is not honesty, the garden plant with its charming, flat, silvery-white, disc-shaped seed pods. Instead, it is a fern. According to folklore, moonwort can open any lock. Hilderic Friend relates the anecdote of a woodpecker mom retrieving a piece of moonwort to open a blocked nest in *Flower Lore.* "They say the Moonewort will doe such things. The experiment may easily be tryed again."[27]

Culpeper suggests that its name derives from its leaf shape, "resembling a half moon."[28] Gerard acknowledges the medicinal uses of the plant, but goes on to report that:

> It hath been used among the Alchymistes and witches to do wonders withall, who say, that it will loose lockes, and make them to fall from the feet of horses that graze where it doth grow ... whereas in truth they are all but drowsie dreams and illusions; but it is singular for wounds as aforesaid.[29]

Ranunculus: This plant is also called buttercup, pilewort, lesser celandine, crowfoot, figwort, smallwort, gold cup, and spearwort. The buttercup family comprises some 400 members. However, crowfoot, or crowflower, derives from its thickened roots, thought to resemble a crow's foot. Culpeper says it's the stalk and leaf shape that gives it that name. Other members of the family (such as the buttercup, the *Ranunculus bulbosus*), have the folk name of "frogsfoot," for the leaf shape as well as the marshy habitat loved by many members of the family. The juice of all members of the family are possessed, to some degree or another, of an irritating, burning quality that herbalists found useful where counterirritants were indicated.

This plant possesses two qualities that land it on Luna's list. First, most of the *Ranunculus* species prefer growing in marshy or wet areas. Second, and more important, is their ability to induce madness, or Luna-cy.

Poor, mad Ophelia drowned herself in a brook, the sodden blossoms draping her body as her most famous icon:

> There with fantastic garlands did she come
> Of crow-flowers, nettles, daisies, and long purples
> That liberal shepherds give a grosser name,
> But our cold maids do dead men's fingers call them . . .
> —*Hamlet*, Act IV, scene vii

Perhaps she inadvertently smelled the "crow-flowers."

The 18th Path: Cancer
Lotus

In denseness, importance, and antiquity, the symbolism of the lotus (*Nymphaea spp.*) is in the same class with the Tree of Life, the bo tree, and the rose. This water plant, with its roots sunk in the muck of the lake-bottom, produces a bloom that ascends upward to the light through the water on a branchless stalk to the surface, there to open to the rays of the Sun. Opening at dawn, it is also famed for closing itself up in the heat of day, when the Sun reaches its height. Mrs. Grieve also notes this disposition in the white pond lily, *Nymphaea odorata*.

Beloved and revered by the ancient Egyptians for food, perfume, medicine, and a symbol of the resurrected soul, the lotus also figured prominently as a sacerdotal offering. Ramesses III once gave over 3400 lotus bouquets to the Temple of Amun.

Turning to ancient Greece, Robert Graves remarks that the golden cup of the Sun, borrowed by Hercules for his journey home after one of his Labors, was lotus-shaped: "This was the cup in which the Sun, after sinking in the West, nightly floated round again to the east along the world-girdling Ocean stream."[30]

The lotus symbolism is congruent throughout cultures worldwide, but it is in the East that the plant's iconography is most fully developed. Each part of the plant—stem, leaf, bud, flower—has its own set of associations. The bud is feminine, the open flower stands for the Sun, and the whole flower is a symbol of beauty, happiness, and eternal renewal. The throne of the gods is a lotus flower. As an attribute, the lotus is depicted mainly with Surya, Vishnu, and Lakshmi (Padma). Vishnu, in particular, is cognate with the lotus. In Sanskrit, the actual word for lotus is *padma*, which is also the name of Vishnu's consort, or *shakti*.[31]

Joseph Campbell suggests that the lotus is the matrix out of which creation manifests, thus earning its position as the pre-eminent symbol of the Great Mother.

In yogic traditions, enlightenment is depicted as the activation of the crown chakra, at or above the top of the head, titled the "thousand-petaled lotus." In Taoism, the same idea is expressed as the "golden blossom" or the "highest lotus." In the Buddhist tradition, of course, the lotus is associated with the Buddha from the moment of his birth. As a newborn, he matured as quickly as Hermes.[32] He literally hit the ground running from his mother's womb. Where his feet touched the ground, lotuses sprang up. The entire iconography surrounding the Buddha is saturated with the lotus in fact or metaphor. The supreme prayer of Tibetan Buddhism, "*Om mani padme hum,*" means "Hail to the gem in the lotus."

The term "lotus-eaters" has come, in the West, to mean languid dreamers, thanks to that tale from the *Odyssey* and Tennyson's poem "The Lotus-Eaters." However, the "lotus" involved was actually the (supposed) narcotic fruit of the lote-tree, a tree whose flowers resemble the lotus. They both belong to the magnolia family. Theophrastus uses the lotus as an example of the frequent difficulty in plant identification. Interestingly enough, the seeds of the lote-tree are used in traditional Chinese medicine as a sedative.

Chapter Eight

The Plants of the Kingdom
and the Four Elements

Malkuth: The Kingdom
Path 32 (*bis*), Earth: Willow, Ivy, Lily
The 31st Path, Fire: Red Poppy, Hibiscus, Nettle
23rd Path: Water: Lotus, and all water plants
11th Path, Air: Aspen

Fire, Water, Air and Earth;
and the Quintessence, Spirit, Informing Them All.

*"Shes a rich girl/ She dont try to hide it/
Diamonds on the soles of her shoes."* —Paul Simon

Continuing our descent on the Tree of Life, we at last come to the final sephira, Malkuth, the Kingdom, the planet Earth. She is the bride of the spirit. For the ancient Qabalist, no single element is attributed to Malkuth. Instead, the Earth sephira is composed of the four elements (Fire, Air, Water, and Earth). These are depicted as the four pie-like slices shown in the diagram of the Tree of Life. Each slice represents one element. At the same time, three paths on the Tree are specifically attributed to three of the four elements (Fire, Air, and Water). There is no path attributed to fourth element, Earth. In our survey of 777's plants, we must accommodate the reality of our existence both as students of Qabala and as magicians. The element of Earth was considered implicit both in Saturn's different instances on the Tree, and in the fact of our living in, through, and on matter. You'd think it would be unavoidable; but Paul Simon's song, quoted below, expresses the problem with precision:

> She said you've taken me for granted
> Because I please you
> Wearing these diamonds[1]

Earth is easily the most misunderstood of any of the four elements. It is the most familiar, and therefore engenders a certain contempt in ways both subliminal and overtly philosophic. We tend to take our good Earth for granted; it is, after all, the ground of our existence. If we start to question it, we'll never even get across the room.

Furthermore, our species demonstrates a real ambiguity when it comes to Earth, to matter. We actually seem to find a kind of comfort in those tired old dualistic theologies. It's not really "comfort," of course, as much as denial, or a false sense of "safety." It is a need brought on, perhaps, by the existential fear of hurtling through vast space at about 67,000 miles per hour. At the same time, the atomic particles comprising the body's most basic level are doing exactly same thing. And each one of this incalculable number is composed mainly of space. Each is, itself, a universe: *That which is above is like that which is below.*

After all that, we just die. Who doesn't want safety, the assurance of some type of "survival" or "transcendence" or, in New Age argot, "ascension"? This beautiful blue planet isn't even good enough to hail from. I've been informed, for instance, by someone who apparently knows, that I'm really a Venusian. The woman enlightening me was herself originally a Pleiadian. And besides, we're going to raise our vibrations so high that we ultimately won't need this embarrassing Earth plane on which our consciousness rides any more. Just a few more years of vegetarianism, or fasting, or celibacy. Just one more round of colonics and that'll do it—you'll see.

The thing is, there isn't really any other "where" to go. To the Qabalist, the Four Elements reflect the Four Worlds of manifestation: Atziluth, the Archetypal World, relates to Fire; Briah, the Creative World, to Water; Yetzirah, the Formative World, to Air; and Assiah, the Material World, to Earth. We find the Four Elements in the *Emerald Tablet*'s formula, distilling our reality's composition:

> *The father of that One Only Thing is the Sun;*
> *Its mother is the Moon; the wind carries it in*
> *its wings; but its nurse is Spirituous Earth.*[2]

Please notice: *its nurse is Spiritous Earth.* Not Earth denied, shut away from shame, salted and ploughed under. This is Earth embraced for the mystery that it is, the mystery of our incarnation, immortal spirit within mortal flesh. In *Angels, Gods and Demons of the New Millenium*, Lon Milo DuQuette writes:

> The Earth in Verse Three [of the Emerald Tablet] is further designated "spirituous" as if to underscore the living presence of the Universal Agent, even in the depth of the lowest elemental world.[3]

Crowley writes that every presentation of the Ace of Disks, *neé* Coins, by every writer up to Éliphas Lévi, is, at best, unsatisfactory and, at worst, villainous. That is why he had to redesign this Ace and rename the suit:

> ... the old conception of the Earth as a passive, immobile, even dead, even "evil" element, had to go. ... Nor are the Disks any more to be considered as Coins; the Disk is a whirling emblem. Naturally so; since it is now known that every Star, every true Planet, is a whirling sphere. The Atom, again, is no more the hard, intractable, dead particle of Dalton, but a system of whirling forces, comparable to the Solar Hierarchy itself.[4]

Astrologers, too, know that the element Earth presents a coalescence of meanings. In birth charts that lack Earth, natives commonly compensate with one of two extremes. Either they live in a world of their own devising—which contacts consensual reality only where unavoidable—or they are compulsively obsessed with the most tedious of trivia, numbering twigs and leaves while the majesty of the forest is lost to them. Robert Hand writes in *Horoscope Symbols*:

> No matter how bound up in fantasies, ideals, or abstractions we are, we must always deal with earth and its concerns. Earth is the ultimate arena in which the acts we perform become manifest.[5]

In other words, it is only "here" that anything happens, anything is real, that the Will, the idea in the mind of God, can be completed. An Arabic version of a verse of the Emerald Tablet states that "*It ascends from the earth to the heaven and becomes ruler over that which is above and that which is below.*"[6] This may serve as a reminder that only after lightning strikes the ground is the flash actually visible. But this verse more commonly reflects the concept shown in Fulcanelli's translation: "*It arises from the earth and descends from heaven; it gathers to itself the strength of things above and things below.*"[7]

The Earth, our reality, is the proving-ground of all ideas, philosophies, theologies, categories, and theories. As the late Sun Bear so often said: "If your philosophy doesn't grow corn, I'm not interested." Earth, the most misunderstood element, grows the corn, provides the support for the theory, nurtures the idea, and substantiates the talk. In *The Marriage of Heaven and Hell*, William Blake has the Devil (Lord and creator of this Earth, to the old Gnostics) say:

But first the notion that man has a body
distinct from his soul, is to be expunged; this
I shall do, by printing in the infernal method, by
corrosives, which in Hell are salutary and medicinal,
melting apparent surfaces away, and
displaying the infinite which was hid.
If the doors of perception were cleansed
Everything would appear to man as it is,
Infinite—
For man has closed himself up, till he sees
All things thro' narrow chinks of his cavern.[8]

Malkuth and Path 32 (*bis*), Earth:
Willow, Lily, Ivy, Oak, [N.B. also Cereals, Pomegranate]

Discussing the various plants attributed to Earth, Crowley writes:

> The Willow is the traditional tree of the neglected maiden, Malkuth
> unredeemed. The Lily suggests that maiden's purity, and the Ivy her
> clinging and flexible nature. All Cereals pertain to Malkuth, Wheat
> being the foundation of the Pentacle which represents Nephesch. The
> Pomegranate is sacred to Proserpine; in appearance also it is strongly
> suggestive of the feminine symbol.[9]

In the note to Path 32 (*bis*), he writes, "The Oak is given on
account of its stability, and the Ivy because of the analogy of Earth
with Malkuth. . . . "[10]

We find further illumination in his description of the Princess of
Disks, in *The Book of Thoth*:

> [She] represents the earthy part of earth. She is consequently on the
> brink of transfiguration. She is strong and beautiful, with an expres-
> sion of intense brooding, as if about to become aware of secret won-
> der. . . . She stands ... before an altar suggesting a wheatsheaf, for she
> is a priestess of Demeter.[11]

Oak: Crowley mentions the oak "on account of its stability," along
with the aspen, the plant given to air, which it "resembles ... by its
trembling." We have addressed the oak in connection with Jupiter and
Mars, but it deserves another glance through this lens of Malkuth. In
The Mystical Qabalah, Dion Fortune writes: "The great point to

remember in connection with Malkuth is that herein is achieved stability. It is in the inertia of Malkuth that its virtue lies."[12] This is the superficial reason why earthquakes are so terrifying.

Willow: The real tree of Malkuth, however, is not the upright and sturdy oak of the Sky Father or the shield tree of the Warrior; it is the graceful, water-loving willow (*Salix alba*). This tree has long and densely saturated associations with goddess lore and women's magick, even without the now-suspect etymology of the word "Wicca." It is a tree linked with the Underworld and with death. The willow was often planted in cemeteries, and is seen at the entrances of the Underworld in Homer, as well as in the sacred black poplar grove of Hecate of the Torches.

The symbolism, however, becomes ambiguous when tempered with the fact of willow's well-known ability to renew itself easily from a twig. Thus it is a symbol of resurrection as well. More evidence of willow being a plant of resurrection is that willow tea (in addition to being, literally, the aspirin of the ancients), has long been used by gardeners as a simple rooting hormone. You want a cutting to develop roots? Soak it in a strong willow tea.

Willow has a weak wood ill-suited for large building projects. However, Hageneder notes that the objects traditionally made from willow are vessels and containers—cradles, coffins, wattle walls, fences, and baskets. All these are for receiving, in symbolic language, the archetypal feminine quality. There is another aspect of willow pointing us toward Malkuth the Bride. Her tree loves water, always the emblem of the Divine Feminine.

We are beginning to see some of the layers of meaning behind the occult truths concerning Malkuth and Yesod. Our physical bodies represent Malkuth, the Earth Kingdom in which we live and move and have our being. Furthermore, we are containers for the forces of Yesod, the Moon, the Mother, ruling the stomach and womb and all water here on Earth. We are composed of about 60% water, thus we respond as much to the Moon's pull as water anywhere. All these notions are woven deftly into the willow.

In Western civilization, as Crowley notes above, the willow is "the traditional tree of the neglected maiden, Malkuth unredeemed." This legacy comes from Psalm 137 in the Bible, where, by the waters of Babylon, the exiled and unredeemed children of Israel weep, remembering their lost Zion, and hang their harps on the willows.

Ivy: Developing his Qabalistic theme of the Maiden, Crowley introduces the "clinging and flexible nature" of ivy (*Hedera spp.*) and thereby agrees with Cirlot that ivy is a feminine symbol denoting the need for protection. Clinging and flexible it may be, but the ivy can kill. Steve Blamires, in his *Celtic Tree Mysteries*, writes:

> The importance of the ivy ... is that, although it seems to be very similar to the vine, it is actually stronger; the vine rarely kills its host, but the ivy, more often than not, does ... even the mighty oak.... Its ability to bind together the trees of the forest and create dense, impenetrable thickets give it an air of malice.[13]

Ivy is an evergreen, and these always imply immortality, even when in need of protection. The Phrygian worshippers of the dying/resurrecting god Attis tattooed themselves with an ivy motif. Needing no protection (*au contraire!*) were the Mænads, the followers of Dionysus. These bands of raving women each carried his *thyrsus*— a staff made of the stalk of the giant fennel, wreathed with ivy and topped with a phallic pine cone. The best advice to those in their path was generally and quickly to get out of Dodge. The ivy was thought to belong to Osiris, reckoned to be the Egyptian Dionysus (or vice-versa). All of these images signify the flow of vegetation and of life. The ivy— evergreen, clinging tenaciously to life, even thriving exuberantly in deepest, driest shade.

Cereals: The Irish word for ivy, *Gort*, means "field," the implications being that of "standing corn." Such an association brings us to the next group of plants, the grains. Crowley relates cereals to the Nephesh, the animal soul and the physical being, which is supported by grains. Crowley invokes (as it were) Demeter in his description of the Princess of Disks, quoted above. But Pamela Berger, writing in *The Goddess Obscured*, observes that the Greek grain goddess, Demeter, is only a shadow of the earlier great vegetation goddess.

The Grain Goddess' critical importance is demonstrated throughout ancient civilizations. In Sumer, for instance, only the king's ritual mating with the Geat Goddess of vegetation ensured the fertility of the land and his continued reign. We find this same ritual explained in terms of our psyche's attaining individuation and integration in Lon Milo DuQuette's *Understanding Aleister Crowley's Thoth Tarot*, where it is told in the form of a Qabalistic fairy tale. The marriage/awakening/redemption of the Princess to her brother, the Prince, results in their assumption of the thrones of their mother and father. The identity of Demeter, Queen of the Fertile Earth, with Persephone, her daughter, Queen of the Realm of Death, is suggestive. The Eleusinian mysteries were founded to commemorate Demeter's search for her abducted daughter. The mysteries promised initiates that they would not join the insubstantial shades at death, partaking of a semblance of life only when blood was spilled for them. Rather, initiates would be blessed in the afterlife, and would remember. Only a queen of the living Earth, as well as a queen of the realms of the dead, would be able to offer and make good such a promise.

Pomegranate: Crowley mentions the pomegranate (*Punica granatum*) almost in passing: "The Pomegranate is sacred to Proserpine; in appearance also it is strongly suggestive of the feminine symbol." He later refers to it as "a symbol with reference to menstruation."[14]

The pomegranate is also a death symbol. We will recall that it was not solely the sacred plant of Proserpine (Persephone); it originally belonged to Hera, Queen of the Gods. Pausanias writes of Hera's pomegranate (the only fruit grown in her honor), that he "must say nothing, for its story is somewhat of a holy mystery."[15] We can make a couple of surmises. One is that the great multiplicity of seeds, each contained in its own little container of sweet-tart juicy pulp,[16] came to stand for fertility, as the fig did. And like the fig, it came to imply the female pudenda. The other guess has to do with Hera's jealousy of Zeus' latest bastard, Zagreus. She instigated the Titans to tear him apart and eat him, either raw or cooked and served in a cauldron. Young Zagreus (the horned serpent) was saved by his dad, as recounted elsewhere. But where the Titans spilled his blood, the pomegranate arose. It is, of course, in the abduction of Persephone/Proserpine that the pomegranate has its greatest fame.

In *The White Goddess*, Graves details the birth of Attis, son of Nana. This virgin daughter of a river god swallowed the seed of either a ripe almond or a pomegranate. When we recall that the tales of Attis/Adonis, as well as those of Zagreus/Dionysus, are all instances of the dying/resurrecting god theme, we have here even more layerings in the meanings of Malkuth's plants. This "earth business" is deep.

Malkuth is certainly the "tomb" so execrated by the Gnostics, and so reviled by a segment of the New Age community, whose "ascension" off our lovely planet is essential to their spiritual growth. However, the other important theme of Malkuth is her function as a womb. Crowley treats us to his hermeneutics of these two motifs in the Ace of Disks. The same tension between the notion of unclean matter and necessary matrix of life is found in the Judeo-Christian treatment of women. To be fair, the "Judeo" part was merely the most recent opportunistic success of patriarchy's Sky Father and did not originate with the Jews. However, the so-called "sin of Eve" was a ball the early Christian Church could run with, and they're running with it still. Even so, the goddess is undeniable—she slipped back in as either the Shekinah/Sabbath Queen, or as the Blessed Virgin Mary. Mary's iconographic flower is the "Madonna" lily, *Lilium candidum*.

The earthy part of Earth, the Princess of Disks, brings us to the final turn of the key in the lock of Malkuth's secret. She carries a scepter, shown diamond-tipped on the card, "a diamond, the precious stone of Kether, thus symbolizing the birth of the highest and purest light in the deepest and darkest of the elements."[17]

The 31st Path, Fire:
Red Poppy, Hibiscus, Nettle

To astrologers, Fire represents the creative force, the life-force, the will. Fire is the only one of the elements (always excepting the Quintessence or Spirit) that is a process rather than a thing in itself. And as the life-force, that's as it should be. The act of living is, itself, a process, not a thing. In the body, Fire is represented by the heat of the living creature as well as by the blood flowing through it. It is the *Yod* of *Yod He Vau Heh* (יהוה), the Primal Fire of Atziluth, the creative Will. Fire is given to the 31st Path, the path of Shin (ש), the Mother Letter meaning "Fire." The shape of the letter itself, with its three Yod-flames, actually represents the element, and its tarot card is Judgment XX. In *The Chicken Qabalah of Rabbi Lamed Ben Clifford* (blessed be he), Lon DuQuette writes that fire is, "the Fire of *Judgment* . . . the central fire of life—the Holy Spirit—the spark that sustains, and finally consumes and transforms all existence."[18]

It is the nature of Fire to consume, to fuel itself for the action that is its process and mode of being. It cannot do otherwise. Other elements luxuriate in their slow rhythms of ebb and flow, or of lazily riding their thermals, or of simply being. We Fire types must keep moving, at least cognitively. We have no choice. This may be the source of Fire's traditional rulership over "work," seen, for instance, in the Wands of tarot; it's a job, being a Fire sign. Fire's color is red, the "hottest" of all.

Since the red poppy and hibiscus are attributed to Fire, as Crowley notes, "only on account of [their] colour,"[19] let us begin with a brief examination of the color red.

Red ochre, derived from iron oxides in the earth, was a vitally important and sacred color to the ancient peoples. As Marija Gimbutas writes, in *The Language of the Goddess*:

> The caves, crevices and caverns of the earth are natural manifestations of the primordial womb of the Mother. This idea is not Neolithic in origin; it goes back to the Paleolithic, when the narrow passages, oval-shaped areas, clefts, and small cavities of caves are marked or painted entirely in red . . . This red color must have symbolized the color of the Mother's regenerative organs.[20]

The color also recalls the "life blood," gift of the Mother, the blood of menses, the blood shed in childbirth. In *777*'s correspondences for "The Body," blood is given for the 31st path of Fire.

Dr. Bruce Dickson, in *Dawn of Belief*, identifies the use of red pigment as one of the first magical acts of our proto-species. The two defining aspects of early peoples—worship of the Mother Goddess and the magical act—come together in the use of red ocher in Neolithic burial sites. The corpses were formed to preserve a fetal shape and buried in womb-shaped vessels, sprinkled with the red pigments "as a way of restoring to them the 'warm' color of blood and life."

In later epochs, other meanings constellated around the color red. It was associated with fire and the masculine, with gods associated with war, and with war in general. This is perfectly exemplified by the 1915 poem "In Flanders Fields." Red poppy pins are commonly sold on Remembrance Day in commemoration of the blood spilled in World War I. However, red has also retained its association as a female color, bringing in Venus to balance all that Martian symbolism. Red is the emblem of the prostitute. In standard iconography, the Magdalene is portrayed either wearing red or clothed only in her hair, which is generally shown as red-gold. Speaking of working girls, we have this justly famous passage from Revelation 17:4–6:

> . . . and I saw a woman sit upon a scarlet-coloured beast . . . arrayed in purple and scarlet-colour. . . . And upon her forehead was a name written, **Mystery, Babylon The Great, The Mother Of Harlots And Abominations Of The Earth** . . . drunken with the blood of the saints . . .

Red is passion: the red roses of Aphrodite or the blood-red rage of Mars. Red is intensely sexual. The red "apple" busted Adam and Eve right out of Eden (whatever fruit was represented, it came to be thought of as an apple). Red generally gets quite a bum rap: both Set and Loki, gods of misrule, have red as their iconic colors. Human red-heads are seen as passionate, irritable, and unpredictable—but always sexy.

Red Poppy: Returning to our discussion of the herbs of fire, we begin with the red poppy, *Papaver rhoeas*. This is not to be confused with the opium poppy, *Papaver somniferum*. The red poppy does have slight soporific properties, but those derive from constituents other than the narcotic alkaloids abundantly possessed by the opium poppy. The distinction is important. A narcotic would run counter to the enlivening nature of Fire.

Crowley writes:

> The Red Poppy is given in this place only on account of its colour, and the same is true of Hibiscus. All scarlet flowers might be equally well placed here. But the attribution is not very satisfactory, as the nature of flowers in themselves is not usually fiery except as their perfume is a stimulant.[21]

I find myself wondering if his dissatisfaction with the placement of the red poppy as one of the plants belonging to Fire has some other cause. Here are some associations that I believe will not only help illustrate the intriguing association of the red poppy with Fire, but also demonstrate the fluidity and intertwining of symbolic imagery.

The red poppy is known by the names copperose, corn rose, cup-puppy, headwark ("headache"), red weed, field poppy, and cock's comb. "Headache" refers to a condition that can be caused by the scent of corn poppies. Mrs. Grieve writes that corn poppies, "have the peculiar heavy odour of opium when fresh, but becomes [sic] scentless on drying." The petals of the corn poppy are always used fresh, and it was traditional for them to be harvested by children. The petals are used in cooking syrups and as a dye for inks and wines, though she writes that the color is generally "too fugitive to be of use."[22] I trust the reader can discern some aspects of Fire in these descriptions. The statement that only fresh petals are used brings to mind that Fire is the only element existing as a "process," rather than as a tangible material reality like a glass of water or the ocean. Thus Fire is either "fresh" or it does not exist at all. Its unpredictable, ephemeral flames could well be described as "fugitive."

Pliny also brings up a very important point about the field Poppy:

> [It is] known to the Greeks by the name of "rhœas".... This last
> grows spontaneously, but in fields, more particularly, which have
> been sown with barley: it ... grows to the height of a cubit, and
> bears a red flower, which quickly fades; it is to this flower that it is
> indebted for its Greek name.[23]

This is a fascinating and rich association, because the "rhoeas" to
which he refers is the pomegranate. In Greek, *rhoa* means red or crimson and signifies the pomegranate. There is an iconographic identity
between the poppy and the pomegranate. As previously mentioned,
the shape of the seed head of any poppy is a fairly exact smaller replica
of that of the pomegranate. The symbolism is the fecundity contained
within the seeds in the womb.

Here, we discover a relationship among the three plants most
closely cognate with Demeter—grain (in this case, barley), the poppy,
and the pomegranate—the three-fold emblem of Demeter as queen of
the Eleusinian mysteries:

> The Eleusinian symbolism of corn [barley], pomegranates and pop-
> pies ... refers to the unseen forces which affect mankind via the veg-
> etable kingdom, building the body and informing the mind.[24]

Demeter is a somewhat kinder and gentler version of the Great
Mother, to whom the poppy was always sacred, signifying as it does
womb and tomb, birth (fecundity) and death (forgetfulness). The
Great Mother is the primordial mother and creatrix, the source of all.
In Erich Neuman's *The Great Mother: an Analysis of the Archetype*,
we begin to become aware of the symbolic association of Fire and the
goddess:

> Like all primordial mothers, she is, in the mythical paradox, her
> father's mother and her son's daughter; that is to say, she bears the
> male by whom she is begotten. She is the vulture Mother goddess ...
> who is worshipped as a "form of the primeval abyss which brought
> forth the light," and whose name means "the father of fathers, the
> mother of mothers, who hath existed from the beginning and is the
> creatrix of the world."... But the goddess is not merely the vessel of
> the Great Round; she is also the dynamic of the life contained in it.
> In Egypt as in India and in alchemy this dynamic is manifested as fire

and heat. This fire can be consuming and destructive, but it can also be the positive fire of transformation.[25]

Later, Neumann discusses what he calls the center of the primordial mysteries of the feminine: namely, "the guarding and tending of fire, . . . female domination is symbolized in its center, the fireplace, the seat of warmth and food preparation, the 'hearth,' which is also the original altar."[26]

Fire resides in the feminine, and is only "called forth" by the masculine, whether by the friction of the sexual act or the action of the fireboard. Agni, the Indian Fire god, is called "he who swells in the mother (the fire board)." The sons of the Great Goddess are light and fire: Light, the "higher," and Fire, the "lower" of the two. Of the four elements, Fire is considered to be nearest to Spirit, embodying (albeit in a "fugitive" and transitory way) the nature of Spirit in a way humans can understand. Thus Zoroaster worshipped Fire as representing the "good" god. Pythagoras taught that Fire's symbol is the triangle, the geometric figure of the divine. We are given "almond in flower" as a secondary plant for the 31st path; this is the plant of Kether, the most exalted sphere on the Tree of Life. And the goddesses Demeter and Hekate are both depicted carrying torches to signify that they own and wield the Fire.

I hope that this brief mythographic excursion into Fire and its correlation with the red poppy, cereals, the pomegranate, the Eleusinian mysteries, and the torches of the goddess might have interested even Brother Crowley.

Hibiscus: The hibiscus named on this list is most probably either the *Hibiscus sabdariffa* or *H. rosa-sinensis,* both members of the *Malvaceae* family, which we met on the 16th path when discussing mallow. After much research, I can only affirm Crowley's statement that it is on this path "only on account of [its] colour." The *Hibiscus sabdariffa* is also known as red tea, roselle, and red sorrel (so called for the sharp, pleasingly acrid taste, similar to sorrel, of its calices—the fruit pods). While its flowers are typically yellow or white, its seed pods are a brilliant crimson, and have been used, dried, as a dye. If you've ever had red zinger tea, you've tasted this hibiscus. It is native to tropical Asia, was introduced into Africa, then into England in the 16th century, and thence to Jamaica, where it enjoys pride of place in the island's cuisine and is a folk-medicine staple. It has a very high concentration of iron (not suprisingly), along with Vitamin C and other vitamins. However, it is important to note that not all hibiscuses are edible—the whole of *H. sabdariffa* is, as is the *Hibiscus rosa-sinensis*, but some of the 300+ members of the family are toxic.

Regarding Nettle, please refer to the discussion in chapter 3, pp. 36–37.

The 23rd Path, Water:
Lotus, and all water plants

Since we have already spent some time discussing the lotus, and "all water plants" is self-explanatory, it is time to turn to an investigation of water itself.

For most Qabalists, as well as for magicians and other workers in the mantic arts, the next element to consider after Fire is Water. Fire is the father, as Water is the mother:

> I am that soundless, boundless, bitter sea.
> All tides are mine, and answer unto me.
> Tides of the airs, tides of the inner earth;
> The secret, silent tides of death and birth.
> Tides of men's souls, and dreams, and destiny—
> Isis Veiled, and Ea, Binah, Ge.[27]

For magicians and astrologers alike, Water is the passive, receptive, magnetic element. Water acts as a physical Akashic record; it receives and holds all the energies exposed to it. This natural receptivity is the source of the psychic ability so often found in Water folk, and also of their infamous moodiness—those tides that Dion Fortune described are always moving. Water relates to Binah, the Creative World, the realm inhabited by magicians when they are committing acts of magick. Water "is" the Hebrew letter *Mem*, and both "are" the tarot card The Hanged Man XII. Rabbi Lamed Ben Clifford (Lon Duquette) has written of Water that it "is the Great Sea—the universal menstrum that carries the vital essence of life (the Blood of Life)."[28]

The race memory of this essence of Water is found today in the blessing of baptismal water on Holy Saturday[29] (the Easter vigil). The priest is creating all the holy water that will be used in his church in the coming year for baptisms, asperging, anointing, and in the fonts. We join the ritual at the point when the Pascal candle has been lit by "new fire," and the priest is exorcising the water:

By the power of the Holy Spirit give to this water the grace of your
Son, so that in the sacrament of baptism all those whom you have
created in your likeness may be cleansed from sin and rise to a new
birth of innocence by water and the Holy Spirit.[30]

Before continuing, the celebrant pauses and touches the water
with his right hand, or he may dip the bottom of the candle into the
water once or three times, then hold it there for the remainder of the
blessing.

We ask you, Father, with your Son to send the Holy Spirit upon the
waters of this font. May all who are buried with Christ in the death
of baptism rise also with him to newness of life.[31]

Not even several centuries of denying the powers of magick can
erase the Church's memory of the nature and power of Water, nor its
relationship with Fire. I leave the analysis of this ritual's symbolism to
the learned reader.

In *Initiation into Hermetics,* Franz Bardon pegs water as well
as any other occult teacher. Bardon describes the more spiritually
advanced characteristics of Water as "humbleness, modesty, absti-
nence, ardency, compassion, tranquility, peace (contentment), forgive-
ness, tenderness." Among the spiritually immature traits, he lists
"indifference, apathy, cold-heartedness, acquiescence, carelessness,
shyness, defiance, inconsistency."[32]

Water people are the sieve though which all emotion, thought, sen-
sation, and feeling pass—or the vessel into which all are poured. They
act from, or toward, whatever has risen to the surface of their consciousness from their unfathomably deep mind, whatever bit of the
pond has flashed silver with the light of the Sun.

11th Path, Air:
Aspen

To the astrologer, Air covers the whole range of mental workings, from
the highest strata of the *Logos* to the week's "scurrilous rags" at the
grocery checkout—from the Thrice-Great Hermes himself to his Ape.
Lon DuQuette writes that *aleph,* the letter of this 11th path, means:

... "ox." In ancient cultures, the ox that pulled the furrowing
plough was a supreme symbol of the fertilizing force of creation.

Aleph is a letter of breath and the closest thing the Hebrew alphabet has to a vowel. As the plough of the ox penetrates and aerates the soil, so the breath of life penetrates and vivifies you and me. Oh hell! I'll come out and say it—the Air of Aleph is more than just the firmament of atmosphere surrounding Earth—it is the Life-Force itself, the Prana of the Hindus, the active ingredient that makes the Holy Spirit holy. Give it some respect![33]

Robert Hand distinguishes the difference between the two masculine elements of Fire and Air. He says that Air is not as unstable, assertive, or willful as Fire. He finds that Air:

shares fire's animated quality. In fact, the word animate is related to words meaning wind. The wind was a metaphor for the soul or spirit because, like them, it animates living matter causing other objects to move while itself is invisible.... [Air] moves about horizontally relating everything it encounters in the physical world to everything else ... [34]

Air is ideas, communication, thought and the faculty of thought, the ability to communicate, and the power of mind all at once. It signifies the birth of the universe and water-cooler gossip, and everything in between. You will not find sentiment among its qualities, nor possessiveness, nor jealousy, nor physical passion. Air comprehends all: truth and falsity are one. The multi-faceted, ever-active, vibratory mind itself is the realm of Air.

Aspen: The aspen, *Populus tremula*, is one of the poplar family. "Populus" means "people" and, like its elemental ruler, Air, the aspen is very happy around people, able to withstand the less salutary effects of civilization like pollution quite well. Aspens will form, after a time, their own society, given that they commonly send up numerous suckers. While this is the reverse of the banyan's process, it still results in a grove or family group. Aspen is said to loosen and revitalize the soil, sharing in the animating qualities of aleph.

The incessant rustling whisper of aspen's serrated leaves on their long, flat stems earns the North American version, *P. tremuloides*, its name "quaking aspen." Folklore attributes this quaking to its being cursed as the Tree of the Crucifixion.[35] But other views suggest that, if the timber had been deemed tougher, harder, more durable, and more valuable, perhaps the legends would have been different. The conceit that aspen wood in unsuitable for use is as unkind as it is untrue—the light, soft, white wood of the aspen resists splintering. During the Middle Ages it was highly desirable for use in the making of shields and arrows.

Aspen has been linked to immortality in various myths. Alder is the fourth tree in the Celtic tree alphabet, *Eadha*. Robert Graves describes alder as "the shifting-leaved white poplar, or aspen, the shield-maker's tree." He recounts how Hercules, after slaying the evil giant, Cacus, bound his head in triumph with white poplar, which he wore when he traveled to and from the Underworld. On his return, "the side of the leaves next to his brow were whitened by the radiant heat he gave out." [36] Thus did Hercules join that select company who were able to make the return trip from the Underworld, and is thereby said to have conquered death.

Another bit of folk legend connecting the aspen and the conquering of death concerns the witches put to death by the Holy [*sic*] Office of the Inquisition. It is said that they were buried in unhallowed ground, and an aspen was laid on the grave to prevent them riding abroad. This is an intriguing, not to say puzzling, assembly of folkloric elements. If aspen is cognate with conquering death, one wonders that it can also be used to deny life after death—or at least the animation of "riding abroad"—to murdered witches. I believe I will invoke the nature of the taboo represented by the aspen, maintaining thereby the identity between the sacred and the damned. Liz and Colin Murray, in their remarkable *Celtic Tree Oracle*, write of the oracular *Eadha* that it has three attributes: an ability to resist and to shield, an association with speech and language, and a close relationship with the winds. *Besoms ready, Grrrrls! We ride tonight!*

PART TWO

The Practice of Herbal Magick

✳

Chapter Nine

PREPARING HERBS FOR MAGICK

Israel Regardie's *Garden of Pomegranates* provides an excellent introduction to the system of classification that seems to have originated with Éliphas Lévi, was elaborated upon by Macgregor Mathers and the rest of the members of the Golden Dawn, and published by Aleister Crowley in 777. Dion Fortune's letter, quoted earlier, implies that Crowley did not make many changes to the Golden Dawn's list of Qabalistic plant correspondences. I believe he was actually reproducing the list from the old Golden Dawn *Knowledge Lectures*. I only have my intuition to guide me, since I am not a member of any of the neo-Golden-Dawn-flavored orders and cannot access their teachings. However, a brief email exchange with someone in the particular G∴D∴ order possessing Fortune's letter informed me that only Qabalistic incense correspondences are taught as part of their Outer Order curriculum. There is nothing taught about the plant correspondences.

Whether this is accurate or not, I cannot say. However, since you are reading this book, you are obviously interested in the magical use of plants. Since I am writing this book, I obviously not only share your interest, but have done quite a bit of work in this area.

There are, of course, a number of ways for the operator to use herbs to enhance magical work. The main considerations are:

1. How dexterous or interested are you at "crafting"?

2. What degree of involvement with the process will satisfy you personally and magically?

3. How much time (i.e., personal energy) or money do you have to devote to the process? (Hint: It's not the money.)

It is always best to be as realistic about these considerations as you possibly can. If you already have a bounteous herb garden, then certainly mixing potpourri and making sachets are already well within your grasp and, depending on the season, may be just a few feet away. If you are either excessively ambitious or obsessive/compulsive, you may want to investigate the art of the stillroom[1] for making your own herbal tinctures, waters, or even essential oils. If even tying your shoelaces is sometimes beyond you, then perhaps candle-dipping is not for you—but rolling beeswax sheets around wicking certainly may be. It is important to be honest with yourself about your skills, your ambition, and your limitations.

Please note: I use the words "herb" and "plant" interchangeably. If I write "flower," I'm referring to the inflorescence produced by the plant.

Let's begin by looking at a few of the basic ways of crafting for the Craft.

Equipment

Your mind, attention, focus, awareness, and consciousness are really your only magical tools. Everything else is only a trigger, a link, a connection between some aspect of your deep mind (*below*), with its source in consciousness itself (*above*). Remember Agrippa's remarks, quoted early in this work: touch any part of the Great Chain of Being "and the whole doth presently shake." Crowley wrote that he once worked magick in the desert with a tin cup for his chalice and a pocketknife for his blade, because all he really needed was his mind.

With that said, let's have a look at the practical tools the magician needs to work with herbs.

Containers: Storage containers should be made of dark glass. Infusion containers should be of clear glass. You can find inexpensively priced canning jars at garage sales. Buy new lids for them at the grocer's. Your local craft store is a source for corks, which can be cut to size, as well as bottles in a variety of shapes and sizes. Clean and dry your supplies thoroughly before use. Welcome them into your life; they will be part of your magical panoply and are worthy of your respect and attention. Avoid plastic and vinyl; they absorb the fragrances. Enamel basins and glass or glazed pottery bowls are very useful to have. You may also consider picking up some big covered jugs and crocks. Some potpourri crafters use metal containers and utensils, but I'm not so sure I would. Your degree of involvement in this process, not to mention the projects you choose, will determine how much equipment you need.

Mortars and pestles: It is essential to have at least two mortar-and-pestle sets—one for harmless plants, one for the toxic. And make sure they are **very clearly labeled.** Wood is not recommended for a mortar.

Stick with marble or glass that won't absorb the plant juices. Suri-bachis, the Japanese mortars, are great for grinding herbs finely. They are used with wooden pestles, so you probably want several of the pestles, clearly inscribed with your (indelible) pen of Art. Clean the Suri-bachi afterward with a stiff brush (again, two cleaning brushes, labeled and kept only for these purposes). While there is a certain tradition suggesting that your tools should be ordinary household things and kept with them, in this particular case, it's not a good idea. You do not want to scrub the henbane out of your "toxics" mortar with the brush you then use to clean your salad bowl (trust me on this).

Grinders: You may find it useful to pick up, again at garage sales, a coffee grinder (or two, see above). The best way to clean these after use is to grind a couple of tablespoons of rice, which will absorb the plant oils. Label carefully as suggested above. Belladonna-infused coffee—I don't think so.

Measuring utensils: Measuring cups and spoons are essential. You will also need an eyedropper for measuring out your ingredients. Non-reactive utensils should be used for stirring, etc. Vinyl works well here.

Protective clothing: You will need to wear rubber or disposable vinyl gloves for certain plants. Even with the innocuous herbs, do you really want to go around smelling like moly all day? There will be times when you'll want to run your bare fingers through your herbs (with some obvious exceptions) to connect with them, communicate the program, and infuse them magically or otherwise energetically. Invoke common sense.

Workspace

In an ideal world, we'd all have "small-c" craft workrooms for our "big-C" Craft projects; unhappily, that's generally not the case. That being said, your kitchen will become both your workroom and your temple. Make sure it is clean before you start your project. You may wish to begin with whatever you're used to doing to establish a sacred space (a banishing ritual, or smudging, if that's what you normally do). A lit candle and incense of the appropriate fragrance[2] will remind you of your magical intention and help you maintain focus. Anything else that will help keep you mindful is all to the good. Make your herbal work a meditation. Ideally, your entire life should be a meditation—how much more so your Magical Work.

Chapter Ten

On Gardening

Gardening is really a luxury and only an adjunct to using plants ritually. That said, there is tremendous satisfaction in going into your own garden; whether you have an actual yard to plant in, or a few pots in a sunny window or under grow-lights, gathering what you need when it needs to be gathered—priceless. All but one of the planets/elements in the magical alphabet have at least one plant suitable for container-growing.

Saturn: Orchis root is but an orchid; dwarf cypresses will grace your terrace.

Jupiter: Anything labeled *ficus* is a fig; shamrock (oxalis) is a common houseplant.

Mars: Red geraniums make a lovely summer hanging basket; cacti, a dish garden.

The Sun: The bay tree makes a handsome houseplant and gives you fresh leaves for cooking. Heliotrope will do fine as a potted plant, too.

Venus: None, alas, of the miniature roses are fragrant, but many of the smaller, old garden roses will do well in pots if their other needs are met. Aloe vera in a pot next to your stove is not only magickal, but practical as well.

Mercury: Marjoram is a favorite "windowsill" herb for pinching off and adding to soups, etc. Potted palms are inexpensive and available at many nurseries. Vervain—like almost any herb—can be container-grown if you give it enough light. While the plant Homer calls moly remains unidentified, there are bulbs of the little yellow ornamental onion with that name that are lovely in a pot with other spring bulbs like narcissus.[1]

Luna: See sources for plants of *Mandragora autumnalis* in the Appendix, p. 115. Give this herb a nice deep pot and do not disturb the root! Mugwort will grow happily in a pot. Just don't take your eyes off it lest it escape, and don't over-water. As a rule, water the silvery plants from below. Potted ranunculus is easily found, especially in the spring; look for plants called "Persian buttercup," or buy the corms in the fall for potting up. Plan a spring dish garden featuring it, moly, and *Narcissus Poeticus.*

Malkuth, and Earth: Potted ivy abounds; the white "Madonna" lily is always sold near Easter, but you can buy bulbs in the fall. There's a stunning new ornamental millet named "Purple Majesty" that grows perhaps three feet tall, just made for container planting. There's a dwarf pomegranate, *Punica granatum var. "Nana."* that grows between four and eight feet tall, and also a dwarf pussywillow of a weeping form (*Salix caprea "pendula"*) that satisfies Crowley's designation of willow as "the neglected maiden, Malkuth unredeemed." Either of these is suitable for a large container (start the young plants off in a gallon pot; repot as needed).

Fire: A hibiscus with edible flowers is *Hibiscus rosa-sinensis,* or Chinese hibiscus, also known as China rose or Rose of China. You'll have to make sure the plant you buy blooms in the appropriate color, because this species blooms red, purple-red, or orange. They are all tender perennials and should only be planted outdoors if you live in a frost-free area.

Water: A whisky half-barrel and a terrace are all you need to get started in water gardening; anything you grow in there belongs to the element of Water. Don't forget a koi or two! Water lilies, a clump of miniature papyrus, maybe a dwarf canna, and you're in business.

Air: Unfortunately, aspen is only suitable for a large yard. I should have guessed that trying to confine the plant belonging to Air in a container was futile. Alternatively, gather aspen leaves and twigs to have on hand when needed. Even better, use Franz Bardon's instructions, discussed in chapter 12, p. 108, to make a simple fluid condenser from them.

Chapter Eleven

The Techniques of Herbal Magick

Important safety note: Exercise common sense, not to mention respect, in all your dealings with plants. Some of them will bite (nettles, cactus, thistle). Some are deadly poison and best avoided altogether (*Strychnos nux-vomica*, many of the nightshades). Some are toxic allergens (rue, wormwood) and some are merely illegal (*Papaver somniferum*, Indian hemp). It is ill-advised, to say the least, to make up an altar potpourri of poisonous plants; even the merely spiky ones require gloves to handle without regret. There are so many physically harmless, but magically potent, plants that you do not need to endanger yourself with the dangerous ones. Choose to be the Magus or High Priestess, not the Fool.

Crowns and Garlands

These are certainly one of the most basic and elemental uses of plants, dating far back into antiquity. Éliphas Lévi incorporates them as integral ritual components described in his books *Transcendental Magic* and *The Magical Ritual of the Sanctum Regnum*. No muss, not much fuss; you will have to know how to put together a simple garland (or swag) and its smaller version, a crown. The only thing simpler would be either to scatter a few of the plants onto your altar and around its base, or to put one plant or a mix of plants appropriate to the working into a bowl of the appropriate color or material as an altar decoration. There's nothing wrong with either of those approaches.

A lovely idea, halfway between your basic pile o'plants and a garland is a mini-garland for your candles. Use *bobéches* at the base of your candles and secure tiny bits of your plants—small leaves, petals, seeds—around them. If you don't want to glue them down, you can use a sticky wax designed to hold candles in place. For example, for a working of Mars, use tiny oak leaves and acorns; for Venus, "sweetheart" rosebuds (that won't be fragrant without your help, but you can't have everything); or you can craft a mini-wreath for the candle bases.

A garland is an uncoiled wreath; a crown is a small wreath you wear on your head. Using your favorite search engine, plug "garland" or "wreath" into it, and you'll be rewarded with a plethora of instructional Web sites. Additionally, the magazine section of your local bookstore and the bookstore itself will more than likely offer numerous crafting magazines and books. Please consult the Resources and Bibliography section for some I've used.

However much plant material you think you'll need—double it. After almost thirty years of wreath-making, I still find it hard to estimate how much I'll need. And it almost goes without saying that, throughout the whole process of gathering your plant materials and making your garland or crown (as well as in any of your "Craft crafts") you are attempting to bring your consciousness, your magical intention, into alignment with your actions. The whole process of making your craft will ideally be a meditation leading up to the actual ritual. If there are some few hours before your actual work, gently coil the garland(s) up and store them in a plastic bag in a cool place (the refrigerator is ideal). The same goes for a crown.

Potpourri/Sachets/Pillows/Powders/Strewing Herbs

These are all different forms of the same thing. A *potpourri* is an assortment of fragrant herbs, petals, leaves, spices, nuts, woods, and perhaps essential oils. If you are making a potpourri of fresh herbs for your altar, that's all you need. If you wish to keep your potpourri, make it from dried plant parts and add a fixative to hold the scent. A *sachet* is a small dry bundle of herbs; a *pillow* is a large one. A *powder* is the same mixture ground fine and sometimes mixed with talc or cornstarch (for using on the body) or not (for ritual use). *Strewing herbs* are sweet-scented herbs and plants that give up their fragrance when trod upon; they needn't concern us unless we belong to SCA.

A potpourri appropriate to your particular working can be placed either in a small bowl on your altar, or gathered up in small cloth bags of the appropriate colors. To make these bags, all you need are squares of cloth tied with ribbons; no sewing need be involved. You can hang them from the corners of your altar or place them on it. You can fold them in squares of paper, sealed[1] with sealing wax or your Glue Stick of Art. It may be too obvious to need mentioning, but when you're making an herbal or plant mix to go into a sachet or pillow, if you intend to keep it, it needs to be absolutely dry. If you'll be disposing of it after the ritual—always with respect—then fresh plant material is fine.

Fixatives: This is both necessary and problematic. In Margaret Robert's book *Potpourri Making*, she writes:

> ... a fixative is an essential ingredient, as it retards evaporation of the fragrance and blends the ingredients together ... I ... encourage people to make their own fixatives from cheap, readily available ingredients which can be grown in their own gardens. These are (a) the common or garden iris, and (b) citrus peels.[2]

Orris root is a famous perfume and fixative known from antiquity. What I did not know is that any common bearded iris will work. And, not having piles of spare ambergris lying about, I was delighted to read about citrus peels as fixatives—ridiculously available! If you're using iris: cut off the root hairs and leaves; wash and scrub the rhizome of soil and mince or grate while still fresh. Spread these gratings on paper and put in the sun to dry. After drying, if you need it powdered, you can crush or grind it.[3]

Regarding citrus peels, you simply save them each time you eat or use a lemon, grapefruit, orange, mandarin orange, or tangerine. (This will encourage mindful eating.) Wash the fruit well before you peel it, as it has probably been oil-sprayed. Mince the fresh peels (no pith) and dry as described above. If it's cold, wet weather, an oven on "warm" will do; stir the bits often. Both peels and crushed seeds make a fine fixative.

Obviously, you will do your best to maintain focus on your magical intention during any and all parts of the procedure. Be aware of the appropriate planetary times for magical work. You can make your magical intention general ("to aid me in my works of Art") if you are going to be preparing a lot of it to store for future rituals. Later, you can consecrate it more specifically to the nature of your work.

Oils: There are three different types of oil you can use in your manufacture of potpourris and other herbal workings.

Essential oils: These provide the predominant "note" of your potpourri. We, as workers of magick, intend all our endeavors to be authentic, and so I strongly recommend essential or aromatherapy oils to insure that what you've bought is pure. You do not want to use "perfume" oils; they are generally synthetic blends. Essential oils can be expensive. In most cases, however, you will only be using a few drops. Essential oils will not go bad. The oils have a variety of uses.

Any good aromatherapy book will guide you into the realm of diffusers, massage oils, bath additives, etc.

Carrier oils: These are oils that are fairly aroma-free in themselves that will absorb the fragrances of the plants or essential oils you blend into them. Some good ones are sunflower oil, corn oil, cottonseed oil, and jojoba oil. Sweet almond oil is particularly good. Its association with Kether helps keep the energy at the highest level possible. Any oils you buy as "carriers" should be refrigerated after opening.

Infused oils: These are perfect for the careful and frugal occultist. Infused oils are those to which you have imparted a concentrated energy of whatever plant(s) you desire by steeping chopped herbs in the oil over a period of time. I have adapted Margaret Roberts' description of the process:

> Chop, macerate, and if appropriate crush your mix of clean, dry herbs (plants, roots, barks, leaves, flowers, fruits, seeds, twigs, berries, etc), enough to fill 2/3 of a quart bottle. Shake two tablespoons of white wine vinegar into your herbs and fill bottle with carrier oil; seal well. Shake and put in a sunny place. Shake daily. Strain the plant materials out, weekly, using a sieve lined with clean cheesecloth or gauze; being sure to squeeze out all the oil from the herbal mix, and discard the pressed, old herbs. Add another bunch of new herbs, two tablespoons white vinegar, and repeat the process until the desired density of fragrance is obtained. Strain and press one final time; store in airtight dark bottles away from the sun. Will keep indefinitely.[4]

These oils are concentrated plant essences that will serve perfectly well for your magical purposes. You can also impart concentrated energy of quite another sort as you work through the stages of the process, so that their vibrational density and magical focus will be in another league altogether than mere "store-bought" oils.

Salt: This is an essential addition that will absorb moisture from the air and keep the potpourri from drying out, thereby keeping it fragrant. Unrefined rock salt, Kosher salt, and sea salt will all work.

Harvesting plants: As a general rule, you should gather herbs in the morning after the dew has dried. However, you may want to time the harvest astrologically. This can be tricky when the first astrological hour[5] of the day comes too early for the dew to have dried. If your plants are still damp when you get them home, gently shake out as much moisture as you can. Then, and oh so tenderly, blot with paper towels. While you are drying your plants, carefully examine them. Even if the plants are dry, examine them carefully. Remove any insects, dirt, and moldy, damaged, or dead parts you find.

Of course, instead of standing in your rose garden, you may find yourself in your grocer's floral section buying a few long-stemmed roses—oh, say mid-afternoon on a Friday in a Waxing Moon. When you get home, strip the petals and, if you'll be using them fresh, mix them up with a few drops of either your essential oil of roses or the infused rose oil you have previously made. (If you're making dried pot-pourri, add the oil at the end of the process.)

Always remember this: We do what we can, when we can, with what we have. It is critically important to overcome a certain natural inertia— "*when* things are perfect, *then* ... " Things are never "perfect." However, in the realm of consciousness or deep mind, in the most real sense, things are "perfect." That being said: there is a vast difference between a sloppy "good enough" attitude—which will surely be reflected in the outcome of your work—and mindfully and scrupulously working within your budget to the best of your ability to achieve your ends. For example, taking the trouble to make infused oils instead of buying essential oils is a good thing. Believe me, the gods know the difference.

Consonant with the traditional caution against haggling when buying magical tools is one of my teacher's favorite precepts, given by *her* teacher: *Don't be a stingy witch.* Always buy the best you can afford. You can be frugal without being mean—you don't want to deflate your magical purpose.

Fresh herbs are best dried in a shady, well-ventilated place. Try spreading them out on paper for two days undisturbed; on the third day, turn and rearrange them. Continue turning them daily until they are completely dry. Margaret Roberts recommends drying herbs in large, shallow trays lined with paper. Another time-honored way is to hang them in loosely tied bundles upside down from a rack or the ceiling without touching each other. This works especially well with flowers. Once they are thoroughly dried, put them away in airtight containers or use them in your project. Dry your woody-stemmed herbs by hanging them in those mesh bags from the grocer (the ones that held onions or apples). It is best to dry each type of plant separately and, if you are drying many of them, label them or make a chart of where each one is. Another of my teacher's pronouncements, proven oh-so-true, is that "one dried herb looks very much like another."

I keep referring to Margaret Robert's excellent book, and I regret that it is out of print. Go online to a book search service to locate one. There are other equally excellent authors. I highly recommend Phyllis Shaudis, whose two books *Herbal Treasures* and *The Pleasure of Herbs* are two of the most useful books you'll ever buy. Again, and unfortunately so, they are out of print, but readily available from online used-book merchants. Remember, "out of print" does not necessarily mean either "expensive" or "unavailable." You can also check your public library, and don't forget the interlibrary loan process that can bring you a book held in any library in your state.

Mixing potpourri: Experts agree that one big secret to successful potpourri-making is to mix for longer than you think necessary. If desired, don your Disposal Vinyl Gloves of Art. In your big bowl, put *absolutely dry* petals, leaves, and other materials (barks, seeds, berries). Mix as if you're mixing the dry ingredients for bread—plunge your hands in at the bottom of the mix and scoop the center from the bottom upward. Keep scooping until you have all ingredients at a good consistency, then add dry salt and mix as before. Add the fixative and mix. Last, add the essential or infused oil and mix well, stirring and working through the whole heap. Crock, seal well, and allow to steep for a week, at which point you can open your crock, have a good smell, and add more ingredients as desired. Seal and steep for another week. "This maturing process is very important as it gives the potpourri its long-lasting mellowness and beauty."[6]

At this point, if you're still not satisfied with your result, you can add more dried petals and leaves, and more of the oil(s), a little at a time, then re-crock, seal, and let it mellow for another while.

You can see that making dried potpourri takes some planning, since it is not an instant process. If you've made up any traditional incense recipes, like Kernunnos or Abramelin (which are really types of potpourris designed to be burnt on charcoal), it's the same process here. Mix, steep, wait, smell, add more of this or that (if necessary), steep again, repeat until you achieve your desired result.

Moist potpourris: These aren't nearly as decorative as the dry ones and take even more time to make, but if properly stored, they will last years. You can immediately see the virtue of having them on hand to be pulled out when needed. Another virtue of the moist potpourri is that you do not need to have all your ingredients at hand before you begin to make it. Moist potpourri is made in stages, so you only need the flowers, herbs, and other plant materials for the stage you're working on. For a nice-smelling "designer's potpourri," use mainly fragrant petals of flowers, but the heady aroma of herb leaves also makes a nice moist potpourri.

Let's say that you have your current stage's plant requirements. Strip their petals or leaves and let them wilt overnight. After a day or so, take a nonmetallic container (a clean gallon-sized jug is ideal, just as long as it has a nice tight-fitting lid!) and spread an inch or so of the wilted plant materials across the bottom. On top of this, sprinkle a thin layer of a coarsely ground salt, like Kosher salt. You can now sprinkle a small handful of mixed, crushed spices—the medieval quartet of cinnamon, ginger, nutmeg, and cloves would go very well here. Over the spices, add another layer of plant materials. Continue the layering as described until you've used up your current stock of ingredients. Put a weight on top of the mixture and let it steep for a period of time. Two weeks is the minimum and works very well with half a lunar cycle, but you can leave it for as long as four weeks, or an entire lunar cycle or zodiac sign, depending upon your magical intention.

After your layered mix has steeped for a half or whole lunar cycle, remove the weight and stir the plant parfait well. Then add your new layers of wilted flowers or herbs, salt, spices, and again weigh it down and leave it to steep as before. Don't forget to press down well each time! Margaret Roberts writes, "The secret is to keep the petals and salt well pressed together—one could call it 'a pickling of petals'! .... This is the true 'rotten pot.'"[7] Continue this process for as long as you like; it makes quite a good Quarter's project.

You'll soon observe the bubbling and foaming that indicate the workings of fermentation, so don't assume you've done anything wrong. (It helps if you've ever made sauerkraut or half-sour pickles, or even wine; there is a stage where you're just *certain* it's nothing but a rotten, smelly mess. Be steadfast!) Near the end of your last stage of steeping, stir the whole mixture well. If you feel it's too wet, simply pour off some of the liquid and let your jug stand another week or more undisturbed.

Now pour the contents out onto your clean working area; break it up and mix in the essential or infused oil of your primary flower or herb. To every five cups of moist potpourri add one teaspoon of essential oil, or two of infused oil. Throw in more spices—the ones you used before, or any others you fancy. To these five cups of moist potpourri, add up to half a cup of mixed spices. Finally, add your fixative—either the dried citrus peels or the minced dried bearded iris (orris) root. For the five cups of moist potpourri we've been discussing, one and a half cups of fixative will do. Mix well and return to the original jug; cover loosely and let stand undisturbed another one and a half lunar cycles (six weeks). At this point, the moist potpourri is ready to store in an airtight jar. When you need it for magical work, scoop out a pile into an appropriate container and place on your altar; you can return it to its jar after your working. When its fragrance begins to wane, a spritz of water and a few drops of essential or infused oil, well-mixed-in, will restore its aroma.

We're not, of course, making potpourris for fragrance; what we're doing is getting our magical ducks in a row. A potpourri at its simplest can be one plant, fresh or dried, with or without fixative. A potpourri for Saturn can be placed in an older pewter bowl (vintage pewter was manufactured with lead). It can consist of a few dried opium poppy pods and/or thistle heads, with a fixative of orris root and a few drops of cypress oil. Saturn "is" lead, poppy, thistle, roots, cypress, and the quality "dry." All these plant correspondences are derived from 777. As we've said, its list of "Plants, Real and Imaginary" is quite versatile and will provide all you need. However, to branch out (so to speak) from the plants of the Tree, you will certainly want to acquire a copy of Rex Bills' *The Rulership Book*, and probably Mrs. Grieve's book, available online at *www.botanical.com*.

Bath Salts

You will take a ritual bath before your working. Why not incorporate the appropriate essential or infused oil into the salt you use? I'm adapting this recipe from *Crafts for the Spirit*, by Ronni Lundy. Here's her basic recipe:[8]

> Salt, coarse bath or sea salt: 1 cup + 2 tbs.
> Epsom salts: 1 cup + 2 tbs.
> Baking soda: 1 cup + 2 tbs.

She suggests four oils, 10 to 25 drops each. I'm guessing these represent for her the four elements: mugwort for Water (Moon); lemon for Fire (Sun); lavender for Air (Mercury); elemi for Earth (peace), which she calls receptivity salts. You can certainly use her recipe as it stands and it sounds lovely. To customize the bath salts, however, I suggest substituting the planetary herbs of 777 as we've discussed.

Saturn: Instead of the 10 drops of mugwort, substitute 10 of cypress.

Jupiter: Instead of mugwort, use 10 drops of hyssop.

Mars: This is problematic (surprise!) as most of his plants are toxic. Your very best bet is to dry some fresh oak leaves, crumble them up, and mix them in with your bath salts.

Sun: You can use the lemon oil Ms. Lundy suggests, 25 drops of it; but again, you've slid out of 777 and into Culpeper, which is perfectly fine. To stay with 777, an essential oil of heliotrope, sunflower, calendula (marsh marigold, which the Old World grimoires and herbals called "sunflower"), bay, or laurel will work. All but the bay will be rather floral; 10 drops will probably do.

Venus: Rose or myrtle—essential oil, of course, 10 to 20 drops.

Mercury: Your choices of essential oils are marjoram, which has a savory fragrance, or the floral lily and narcissus. I find narcissus cloying, along the same order of hyacinth, so I'd probably go with the marjoram. Ten to 20 drops. (Culpeper has lavender.)

Luna: Put that mugwort back in—10 drops! Or you also have almond, hazel, and lotus to choose from. I'd use 10 of almond and 5 of hazel or lotus.

Malkuth: Again we have the lily, but also the pomegranate.

Fire: Brew up a pot of strong nettle tea, or an infusion of oak leaves. Failing that, here's another example where it would be to your advantage to make infused oils of red poppy (*Papaver rhoeas*) and hibiscus (*Hibiscus rosa-sinensis*). Either can be used without scruple on your skin.

Water: Lotus again, or any water plant

Air: Aspen. Here again is another case for a tea, or even better, an infused oil. I don't think you'll be likely to find a ready-made essential oil of aspen.

Earth: See Saturn or Malkuth.

Candles

There are any number of good Web sites and books that will guide you through the manufacture of your own candles; please see the Resources and Bibliography section for some I've used. The methods run the gamut from simple to goddess-awful messes—at least that's been my experience. It is very gratifying, to be sure, to make your own candles out of melted wax. I have made poured candles (votives and large molded pillars), as well as dipped tapers. These projects require a guide that is really a book in itself. If you choose to go the melted-wax route, Scott Cunningham's *Spell Crafts*[9] has some excellent observations and suggestions about magical candle-making in general, and also about the use of essential oils and herbs, like putting relevant fresh herbs, minced, into your melted wax. However, for our brief guide, I will confine myself to candles that are easy and quick to make and also have a high satisfaction quotient. I'm talking about rolled candles made from sheets of beeswax, though you may use what you will. Beeswax, however, is entirely natural and its own fragrance imparts a lovely honey scent as the candle burns.

You'll need a sheet or two of beeswax in the color(s) you require (see Resources and Bibliography, p. 115) and some wicking. The sheets are usually 8" x 16". While you certainly can make your own wicking,[10] it's best to bite this small bullet, pay the couple of bucks, and buy a pack of tailor-made wicking at your local craft store. The basic technique is this: On a clean surface, with a sharp blade (X-acto or Bolline) cut a *malleable* sheet[11] diagonally into two triangular shapes. Start rolling on the shortest side. Cut wicks an inch or so longer than your finished candle. Make a channel on the short side for the wick (that is, fold up one row of the cells; it will be about a quarter of an inch or so wide) and press the wick firmly into it. Then begin rolling, using an even pressure. Do not rush. If the sheet becomes cold, fire up the hairdryer. When you've rolled it all up, roll it under your palms, back and forth on the flat clean surface to even out the sides (like rolling out clay "snakes"). Press the seam with your fingers to seal; even off the bottom of the candle, if needed, with your blade.

One method I adapted from some bought rolled candles is this: Use the same half-sheet triangle for a candle, but, from another sheet altogether, cut a strip 1" (or more) wide x 16" long. Lay this strip to overlap about one-half inch down the longest side of your triangle. This strip will not be quite as long as the hypotenuse and that's ok. Line the strip up at the base end. When you get to the tip end, fold the little triangle flap at the very top down over it anyway. Roll as usual. You will have to pay particular attention that the strip is well-pressed into your triangle sheet, because it has a mind of its own and it's up to you to make sure it sticks with the program. The simple addition of this strip not only allows you to craft a candle in the Flashing Colors or seasonal colors if desired, but gives a more pleasing overall shape— more tapered, not as conical, and nicely tall.

Another method is simply to roll one candle from the sheet, starting at the 8″ end. If you want a tall candle, you can start on the long side. You can, if you like, add another sheet (or two), overlapping toward the end of your original sheet if you want a fat pillar. A variation is to make four votives from one uncut sheet. Cut the sheet first into 2″ x 16″ pieces, then roll up your votives. The resulting candles will fit nicely into your Quarter lamps.

That's the basic procedure. I'd like to add one additional step. Keep at hand a bowl of very finely chopped (or crushed) and dried magical plants pertinent to the working—leaves, petals, seeds, berries, chips of wood, all fragranced with your essential or infused oil (no fixative needed). As you are rolling your candle, scatter these thinly onto the candle's inside surface, maintaining all the while your magical intention. Finish with your usual candle blessing or dressing. You have the ability to make every part of your preparatory work a meditation and part of your inner work. There's no reason to rush through and cheat yourself of this; after all, the inner work is the "real" magical work, and your outer work will reflect that. If you rush to get to what you consider the "real" magical work, you'll have lost the valuable truth that *it's all magical work. As above, so below; and as below, so above; to the Glory of the One Thing.*

Poppets

The word itself derives from the French or Italian words for "puppet." A poppet, usually a stuffed cloth doll, can stand in for any person (subject) in your magical working, particularly if it carries on or in it something of the subject. This can be a product of the subject's body, a photograph or photocopy of a photograph, a sample of handwriting, or a sketch of the subject's face on the doll recognizable at least to you. When you combine these energetic links from the subject with the herbs appropriate to your working, ritually sealed up in your ritually named poppet, you have an extremely powerful magical tool. You will certainly want to put your poppet through some sort of "naming" ceremony as part of the magical linkage with the subject. I'm certain you have your own preferred rituals for this process, and if you don't, you won't have to look very hard to find one in a book or online. Poppet magick can be used to promote or encourage the subject's protection, healing, love, prosperity, success, study skills, eloquence—in short, any type of spell whatsoever. Note that I've only mentioned some "day-side" applications of poppet magick. My personal experiences demand that I inform you that *the Laws of Karma operate acutely and unexpectedly in this arena, so* **please** *examine scrupulously any proposed spellwork before you act.*

I wish to thank Lisa-Marie Jackson, of Suffolk, England, the "White Witch" of Angelfire, who very kindly gives me permission to use the material from her thorough Web page on poppets.[12] I am adding my own notes, italicized, and hope they augment her fine work. There are various types of materials used to make poppets. Let's consider them in turn.

Wax: Soften candles and shape them into poppet figurine. Rub lavender or similar oil *[I recommend almond: belongs to Cancer, the Mother, and you are, after all, "birthing" this creature]* onto your hands first for ease *[i.e., before you begin the shaping; it will help you manipulate the wax].* Make sure the wax is not too hot. Use small pieces of coal or gems to adorn the poppet. If you desire a more powerful effect use hair, fingernails, or some other token or possession of the recipient.

Since this work deals with plants, gems aren't necessary. Alternatively, a beeswax block bought from a candle-making supply house (or health-food store). Beeswax blocks are kind of expensive, but easier to work with than paraffin, which tends to "shatter." Another possibility is to visit your local brick-and-mortar for supplies. You can visit (in person or online) any Gris-Gris, Root, or Hoo-Doo Shop and purchases a few Figure candles. You'll find them available in black, green, red, pink, white, and brown. Any such Shop worth its High John Root will stock them. With my lack of sculpting skills, the fact that they're pre-formed trumps their lack of beeswax. Of course you would ritually cleanse any candle you've made or purchased before use. With the Bolline or Working Knife, slit the Poppet along its side, or wherever on its "body" you can hollow out a hole for the herbs appropriate to your Work, just a pinch or two, along with any other energetic links. Plug and seal the opening with left-over wax. Proceed with "Naming cermony."

Cloth: Cut round a template on two pieces of cloth, stitch almost all the way up, then fill with herbs, or hair. Adorn with colored threads, or draw symbols. The name of the recipient can be written on the poppet. *[Draw a "gingerbread man" as large as you want your poppet-to-be, being sure to add half an inch for a seam allowance along the edge. Pin your template onto a folded piece of fabric, (so you have two layers—front and back) of cloth of the color appropriate to the work. Cut out and stitch along the perimeter of the poppet, leaving it open along one side, a couple of inches' worth, to allow you to stuff it. Turn the poppet inside-out. Stuff it almost completely full with batting, poking the batting down so it fills the arms, legs, and head evenly. Be sure to leave space for your links and herbs (see above). When filled to your satisfaction, stitch up the open bit of seam. Proceed with decoration (see above) and "naming ceremony."]*

Paper: This is the quickest way. Simply cut paper *[and this may ideally be a sheet of the paper you made yourself (see Resources and Bibliography, p. 115) with the appropriate herbs already incorporated in it]* into poppet figure. You can then anoint with oil and draw symbols on it. You can even glue a photo on it of the person the Poppet is intended to represent. *[If you don't have any homemade paper, since this poppet will take glue easily, you can glue some of the dried herbs appropriate to the work onto it. For instance, a dried sweetheart rosebud at its heart area for a work of Venus.]*

Wood: Carve poppet into figure, glue on hair or use a piece of cloth from the clothing of the recipient of the spell. Use paints or crayons to adorn the poppet. *[Either carve the poppet out of a piece of the appropriate planetary or elemental wood, or (easier) use whatever wood you have, ideally a fairly soft one. Remove a plug, hollow out a small compartment, and fill it with the herbs and energetic links. Replace the plug using your Glue of Art, or melted wax. Paint etc., if desired; continue to the "naming."]*

Root: Several plant roots can be carved into poppet figures such as potato, apple, and ginseng *[also horseradish (wear gloves!), carrot, parsnip, parsley, celeriac. Name as usual.]* Make sure the poppet is finished before using it; do not carry on carving once you start using it. This poppet is for short-term use as it will inevitably rot. *[Well ... it doesn't have to be for the short term, but that's outside the scope of the present work.]*

Clay: Mold into poppet shape; be sure to create a hollow to place hair, fingernails or herbs, etc. before sealing. Adorn with paints or by carving with a sharp object. *[First the decision: earthen clay or synthetic? Agrippa would have you, with your virgin lad holding the lantern, out in the dark digging up earthen clay with your bare hands. We probably don't need to go beyond your local craft store where you can buy a few pounds of earth clay to keep on hand, well-sealed in plastic bags to keep it moist. Form as above; "name" as usual.]*

In modern days, the most common poppets are filled with herbs and incense. But pure Witchcraft still uses the practice of urine, blood, fingernails, and hair *[as well as tears, sweat, semen, or menstrual blood]*.

The poppet will be magically charged by the Witch, using a simple spell, chant, song, dance, drumbeat, or other straightforward method.

Depending on the desired outcome, use the elements, winds, or moon phases to bring life to the magick.

Important: Take really good care of your poppet when not in use. The last thing you want is to accidentally drop it and break it, or set fire to it etc. Wrap it in white cloth *[I use silk cloth of a color appropriate to the work; but certainly white is always acceptable]* and keep it somewhere safe. To dispose of a poppet, dig a deep hole and bury it. Be sure to sever the magical link between the poppet and the person before disposing of it. This information was shared in the good faith that no reader will use this to bring harm to another.[13]

Other Herbal Magick Creations

As I wrote earlier, the only real limit to what you can do with your plants is your imagination. Once you have an idea, plug the concept into your favorite search engine and see what turns up. You'll almost certainly be able to find instructions on how to make it, or be directed somewhere you can find out how. Here are some other miscellaneous good ideas deserving far more space than I'm allotting them.

Handmade paper: I've never made it, and so will not attempt to describe the process. The authors who do always seem to suggest adding bits of dried flower petals or leaves to the pulp. This led me to an instant realization that handmade paper, containing the proper bits of plant stuff and made on the appropriate days, times, etc., would be perfect for use in a magical journal devoted to those workings. There's even an on-line tutorial in bookbinding, so you can bind the journal yourself out of paper you make. Less ambitious, but equally enhancing energetically, are those sachets mentioned earlier. Fold them up in your handmade papers.

Altar cloths, banners, hangings: While you can affix dried flowers[14] and or leaves appropriate to your work on the hem of your altar cloth, etc., the end result will perforce be fragile. However, Laura Martin, one of my favorite gardening writers, developed an entirely new craft she calls "Pounding Flowers."[15] Very basically: With a hammer, pound the flower or leaf onto whatever it is you wish to take the image and actual color of the plant. I hope you can sense the exciting applications this craft has. Buy the book! The one and only *caveat* I would add is this: After you've gathered your materials (plants and cloth, leather, ribbon, etc.), but before you begin pounding away, asperge and bless your hammer, materials, and plants, dedicating them all to your work. Before you begin pounding, address your plants; tell them what you will be doing with them and why. This craft, while brilliant, is admittedly a violent way to transfer a plant's energies to a medium, and your plants deserve at least an explanation and dedication to your work.

Corn dollies: This lovely and ancient craft is resonant with the energies of the Great Corn Mother, with Demeter, with Brigit, with old agricultural festivals—an altogether worthy craft to master and totally appropriate to Malkuth. Legends across cultures have the Grain Spirit fleeing the harvester's scythe until it was trapped in the last handful of corn on the field. This last sheaf was treated with especial care and kept over the winter, for it preserved the spirit of the grain so that the next year's harvest would be bountiful. Of the many ways this sheaf was preserved, the corn dolly—certainly not always a "dolly," but often a stylized cage—was one that kept the Grain Spirit enclosed and safe. If you grew the Purple Majesty millet recommended above, you're all set. Otherwise, use your resources to come up with an appropriate substitute.

Chapter Twelve
Franz Bardon and Herbal Magick

Franz Bardon is an island in the boundless sea of occultism, an occult singularity seldom studied save by his students. Bardon "invented"—as far as anyone can tell—his own intensely interesting system of herbal magick with which he augmented his ritual work. His construction of elemental fluid condensers can easily be adapted as planetary condensers and has immediate application in the ritual charging of talismans. In this use of the condensers, the talisman is moistened with the appropriate fluid condenser and allowed to dry. This method can be assimilated into your regular ritual of talismanic construction and add depth to your work. Bardon describes in detail the entire process in *Initiation into Hermetics*. For further study, please consult this work. Please also note that Bardon's use of the word "fluid" varies from an equivalency to "vibration" or "energy" to the actual liquid.

For Bardon, water is the prime magnetic fluid of importance because of its receptivity. He writes:

> Not only water but all liquids have the specific attribute of attraction and . . . the ability to retain influences, whether good or bad . . . The Water element and especially physical or material water can be regarded as an accumulator. The colder the water is, the greater its capacity to accumulate.[1]

Very simply put, the point of making fluid condensers is to unite Water and appropriate herbs in a ritual manner to accomplish the magician's will.

While Bardon suggests initiates will recognize appropriate plants by their signatures, we are going to stick with our 777 list. Whether the magick is elemental or planetary, all the operator needs to know are the plants, the hours, and the recipe for the fluid (i.e., liquid) condenser.

The one necessary element of any condenser is "a small amount of gold," and, since this can be a homeopathic preparation dissolved in a bit of spring water (use 100 pellets for every cup of water), the operator won't be beggared by the construction of the condensers. (Bardon preferred rainwater, but he was writing in pre-acid-rain days.) Any

homeopathic "brick" or "click" shop will have *Aurum chloratum,
A. muriaticum,* or *A. metallicum.* Since each condenser only needs a
few drops, this will last you quite a long time.

Preparation of a simple fluid condenser: With spring water, cover one
handful of either fresh or dried herb in a nonmetallic, lidded container
(e.g., enamel or tempered glass). Bring to a boil, reduce to simmer, and
continue to simmer, covered, for 20 minutes. Remove from heat
and allow to cool completely, still covered. Filter to remove the herbs
(be sure to press all liquid from them). Place the "tea" in a clean (non-
reactive) pot and simmer uncovered until reduced to a scant quarter of
a cup. Mix in the same amount of alcohol as you have tea (190-proof
grain alcohol or, failing that, vodka) to prevent mold; add about 10
drops of the gold solution. If the condenser will be for your personal
purposes, Bardon recommends adding a bit of your own blood and, if
male, your sperm. Shake well, and filter again. Store your condenser in
a dark-purple bottle, well-sealed in a dark and cool place, ready for
use. A fluid condenser that has been prepared in this manner will not
lose its effectiveness for many years. Before using the condenser, shake
well each time, then seal well after use and continue to store in a cool
dark place.

I've purposely left the herb of this recipe unspecified. Bardon uses
chamomile, an herb always associated with the Sun. I'd use crushed
bay leaves, sunflower, or any other of 777's solar herbs. To change the
magical focus of your condenser, substitute an herb from the list of elements or planets we've discussed, such as hibiscus for Fire, aspen
leaves for Air, etc.[2]

Preparation of the compounded universal fluid condenser: This form
of condenser achieves a greater concentration of energy and is especially useful when the operator wishes to exert a physical influence in
addition to the mental-astral workings of the simple fluid condenser—
for instance, for use in poppet magical workings. The recipe for the
compounded universal fluid condenser combines several different
plants. Bardon gives three different methods of preparation, increasing
in degrees of complexity:

1. For the first method, see above. Take equal amounts (by volume) of the herbs, proceed as above. In the second stage, simmer until
the mixture is as thick as possible without burning or becoming too
dry—you want a thick reduction. Measure this after it has cooled, add
alcohol, etc., just as described above.

2. The second way is the alcohol-tincture method. *This method is the only one you should use* when you are making a condenser of toxic plants like rue, henbane, belladonna, etc. **Take all necessary precautions when working with toxic plants.**

Place equal amounts by volume of the herbs into a glass jar just large enough to hold them, and cover with alcohol. Seal tightly and let macerate for 28 days in a warm place. Then filter carefully by pressing the residue through a linen cloth (gloves!), or muslin, or several layers of cheesecloth, then through a filter paper. Next, measure the herbal liquor and add the gold tincture/solution—one drop for every third of an ounce of the herbal liquor. Add your blood or sperm as before. Bottle and store for your own use.

3. Bardon describes the third method as the best, although it is the most energy- and time-intensive. Prepare each herb individually, as a simple fluid condenser, using either the first or second method. Once you have all the extracts prepared, mix them in equal proportions, add the proper amount of gold tincture/solution, and store in a cool and dark place.

I recommend adding the same ritual considerations that pertain in any other magical operation to the preparation of any fluid condenser. Decide whether your operation, or parts thereof, can/must be performed inside your circle, temple, or other sanctified space. Do you need to make a temporary temple of your kitchen? What would that involve? *Think it through.* Most important, define your magical intention and select your means of focusing on it as you proceed through the operation. Choose the appropriate day, lunar sign and phase, planetary hour, etc., for your operation or a particular stage of the operation. Ritually cleanse and exorcise beforehand your tools, pots, lids, strainers, bottles, etc. (This is not necessary for the herbs. Bless them, of course, and dedicate them to your work. And be sure to wash and dry fresh herbs before you begin.)

Other matters may occur to you. Write them down and figure out beforehand how you will handle them. There's nothing quite like standing in your kitchen with a strainer of dripping herbs, for instance, and realizing that you forgot to buy cheesecloth. And that you have precisely three minutes before the Moon moves out of phase to come up with some substitute. You never really liked that tee-shirt you're wearing, after all!

Afterword

We have arrived at the end of this little book. I have tried to give you some knowledge and direction in an area of magick often neglected by witches, and all but forgotten by ritual magicians. Magical plants and herbs are the living link between our minds and the world in which we live. When we work with them mindfully, they root us in Malkuth and provide us with the stability we need to reach, successfully, for the heavens. The Emerald Tablet teaches us unequivocally that:

> ... *the superior agrees with the inferior, and the inferior with the superior, to effect that one truly wonderful work.*

That herbs are at the "inferior" end of the Great Chain of Being does not mean they are of no consequence. Remember Agrippa's teaching: Touch that Chain at any point and "the whole doth presently shake."

I wish you great joy in your herbal, and all other magical, works!

Resources and Bibliography

The classic must-haves:

Beyerl, Paul. *The Master Book of Herbalism.* Custer, WA: Phoenix Publishing, 1984.

Cunningham, Scott. *Cunningham's Encyclopedia of Magical Herbs.* St. Paul, MN: Llewellyn Publications, 2005.

Huson, Paul. *Mastering Herbalism.* 1977. London: Abacus, 1977.

Hyslop, Jon and Ratcliffe, Paul. *A Folk Herbal.* Oxford: Radiation Publications, 1989.

History

Berger, Pamela. *Goddess Obscured. Transformation of the Grain Protectress from Goddess to Saint.* Boston, MA: Beacon Press, 1985.

Cooke, Mordecai C. *The Seven Sisters of Sleep.* Lincoln, MA: Quarterman Publications, Inc., 1989.

Dickson, D. Bruce. *The Dawn of Belief.* Tucson, AZ: University of Arizona Press, 1990.

Dunand, François and Christiane Zivie-Coche. *Gods and Men in Egypt, 3000 B.C.E. to 39C.E.* Ithaca, NY: Cornell University Press, 2004.

Lawrence, Marilynn. "Hellenistic Astrology," Ch. 2.b, of *"Greek Medicine."* Internet Encyclopedia of Philosophy, *http://www.iep.utm.edu.* This is the home page; I have been unable to access the article from the URL I have, but it can be found via the Index under "Astrology, Hellenistic."

Tester, Jim. *A History of Western Astrology.* Westminster, MD: Ballentine Books, 1989.

Primary Texts

Cashford, Jules, trans. *The Homeric Hymns.* London: Penguin Books, 2003.

Josephus, Flavius. *The Wars of the Jews.* trans. William Whiston, *http://www.perseus.tufts.edu/cgi-bin/ptext?lookup=J.+BJ+7.163*

Pausanius. *Description of Greece with an English Translation by W.H.S. Jones, Litt.D., and H.A. Ormerod, M.A., in 4 Volumes.* 1918. William Heinemann Ltd. *http://www.perseus.tufts.edu/cgi-bin/ptext?lookup=Paus.*

Pliny the Elder. *The Natural History.* trans. and ed. by John Bostock and H.T. Riley. 1855. Taylor and Francis. *http://www.perseus.tufts.edu/cgi-bin/ptext?lookup=Plin.+Nat.*

Magic, Hermetics, Grimoires

Agrippa, Henry Cornelius. *Three Books of Occult Philosophy. Book I.* trans. by James Freake; ed. by Donald Tyson. St. Paul, MN: Llewellyn Publications, 1998.

Bardon, Franz. *Initiation into Hermetics*. Salt Lake City, UT: Merkur Publishing, Inc., 1999.

Cotnoir, Brian. *The Weiser Concise Guide to Alchemy*. San Francisco, CA: Weiser Books, 2006.

Crowley, Aleister. *777 and Other Qabalistic Writings of Aleister Crowley*. ed. by Israel Regardie. New York: Samuel Weiser, Inc., 1979.

Crowley, Aleister, with Evangeline Adams. *General Principles of Astrology*. Weiser Books, 2006.

della Porta, Giambattista. *Natural Magic*. *http://homepages.tscnet.com/ omard1.jportac1.html#Chap38k1*.

DuQuette, Lon Milo. *Angels, Demons & Gods of the New Millennium*. San Francisco, CA: Samuel Weiser Inc., 1997.

_____. *The Chicken Qabalah of Rabbi Lamed Ben Clifford*. San Francisco, CA: Weiser Books, 2001.

_____. *My Life With the Spirits*. San Francisco, CA: Samuel Weiser Inc., 1999.

_____. *Understanding Aleister Crowley's Thoth Tarot*. San Francisco, CA: Weiser Books, 2003.

Ficino, Marsilio. *Three Books on Life*. ed. Carol. V. Kaske; trans John R. Clark. Medieval and Renaissance Texts and Studies, 1998.

Fortune, Dion. Letter to Israel Regardie. Nov. 1st, 1932. Tempe, AZ: Hermetic Order of the Golden Dawn, 1997-2006.

_____. *The Mystical Qabalah*. London and Tunbridge: Ernest Benn Ltd., 1976.

_____. *Sea Priestess*. New York: Samuel Weiser, Inc., 1981.

Lévi, Éliphas. *The Book of Splendours*. Wellingborough: Aquarian Press, 1981.

_____. *The Magical Ritual of the Sanctum Regnum. Interpreted by the Tarot Trumps*. trans. W. Wynn Wescott. Berwick, ME: Ibis Books, 2004.

_____. *Transcendental Magic*. trans. A. E. Waite. San Francisco, CA: Weiser Books, 2001.

Miller, Richard Alan and Iona Miller. *The Magical and Ritual Uses of Perfumes*. Rochester, VT: Destiny Books, 1990.

Pike, Br. Albert. *Morals and Dogma of the Ancient and Accepted Scottish Rite of Freemasonry*. Richmond, VA: L.H. Jenkins, Inc., 1919.

Regardie, Israel. *A Garden of Pomegranates*. St. Paul, MN: Llewellyn Publications, 1970.

Herbals and Herbalism, History and Practice

Culpeper, Nicholas. *Culpeper's Complete Herbal*. Slough, UK: W. Foulsham & Co., Ltd., n.d.

Foley, Daniel J., Ed. *Herbs for Use and for Delight. An Anthology from "The Herbarist," A Publication of the Herb Society of America*. Mineola, NY: Dover Publications, 1974.

Gerard, John. *The Herbal or General History of Plants. Complete 1663 Edition as Revised and Enlarged by Thomas Johnson.* New York: Dover Publications, 1975.

Grieve, Mrs. M. *A Modern Herbal.* Middlesex, UK: Penguin Books, 1977.

Hanson, Harold A. *The Witch's Garden.* trans. Muriel Crofts. Santa Cruz, CA: Unity Press/Michael Kesend, 1978.

Potter, Samuel. *Therapeutics, Materia Medica and Pharmacy (14th ed.).* Revised by R. J. E. Scott. P. York, PA: Blakiston's Son & Co., 1926.

Russo, Ethan. *Handbook of Psychotropic Herbs.* Binghamton, NY: Haworth Herbal Press, 2001.

Schultes, Richard Evans and Albert Hoffman. *Plants of the Gods: Origins of Hallucinogenic Use.* New York: Alfred van der Marck Editions, 1979.

Strehlow, Wighard and Gottfried Hertzka. *Hildegard of Bingen's Medicine.* Santa Fe, NM: Bear & Co., 1987.

Stuart, Malcolm, ed. *The Encyclopedia of Herbs and Herbalism.* London: Orbis Publishing, 1979.

Theophrastus. *Enquiry into Plants.* trans. Arthur Hort. London: Loeb Classical Library, 1999.

Astrology, Tarot, Oracles

Barz, Ellynor. *Gods and Planets.* trans. Boris Matthews. Wilmette, IL: Chiron Publications, 1993.

Bills, Rex. *The Rulership Book.* Richmond, VA: McCoy Publishing & Masonic Supply Co., Inc., 1971.

Crowley, Aleister. *The Book of Thoth.* New York: Samuel Weiser, Inc., 1974.

Forrest., Stephen. *The Inner Sky.* San Diego: ACS Publications, 1988.

Hand, Robert. *Horoscope Symbols.* West Chester, PA: Whitford Press, 1981.

Lilly, William. *Christian Astrology.* Renaissance Astrology, 1647. *http://www.renaissanceAstrology.com/lilly.html.*

Morin, Jean-Baptiste. *Astrological Gallica; Book Twenty-Two.* Tempe, AZ: American Federation of Astrologers, 1994.

Murray, Liz and Colin. *The Celtic Tree Oracle: A System of Divination.* New York: St. Martin's Press, 1988.

Mythology, Psychology, Symbolism, Folklore

Steve Blamires. *Celtic Tree Mysteries.* St. Paul: Llewellyn Publications, 2003.

Campbell, Joseph. *Myths of Light: Eastern Metaphors of the Eternal.* Novato: New World Library, 2003.

Cooper, J. C. *An Illustrated Encyclopedia of Traditional Symbols.* London: Thames & Hudson, 1987.

Frazer, James. *The Golden Bough. The Roots of Religion and Folklore.* New York: Avenel Books, 1981.

Friend, Hilderic. *Flower Lore.* Rockport, MA: Para Research, 1981.

Grigson, Geoffrey. *The Goddess of Love*. New York: Anchor Press, 1978.

Hageneder, Fred. *The Meaning of Trees*. San Francisco, CA: Chronicle Books, 2005.

_____. *The Spirit of Trees*. New York: Continuum, 2005.

Gimbutas, Marija. *The Language of the Goddess*. San Francisco, CA: Harper & Row, 1989.

Godwin, Joseclyn. *Mystery Religions in the Ancient World*. San Francisco, CA: Harper & Row, 1981.

Graves, Robert. *The Greek Myths. Vol. I*. London: Penguin Books, 1975.

_____. *The White Goddess. A Historic Grammar of Poetic Myth*. New York: Farrar, Straus & Giroux, 1981.

Huxley, Aldous. *The Doors of Perception/Heaven and Hell*. New York: Harper & Row, 1990.

Moore, Thomas. *The Planets Within*. Hudson, NY: Lindisfarne Press, 1990.

Neumann, Erich. *The Great Mother: An Analysis of the Archetype*. Princeton, NJ: Princeton University Press, 1974.

Walker, Barbara. *Woman's Dictionary of Symbols and Sacred Objects*. San Francisco: Harper San Francisco, 1988.

Wang, Robert. Personal email to the author, dated Nov. 4, 2005.

Crafts

Cunningham, Scott and David Harrington. *Spell Crafts. Creating Magical Objects*. St. Paul, MN: Llewellyn Publications, 1993.

Jackson, Lisa-Marie. *"Poppets." http://www.angelfire.com/realm/white_witch;* © *White Witch 2001.*

Lundy, Ronni. *Crafts for the Spirit. 30 Beautiful Projects to Enhance Your Personal Journey*. New York: Lark Books, 2003.

Martin, Laura C. *The Art and Craft of Pounding Flowers*. Mt. Kisco, NY: QVC Publishing, 2001.

Oppenheimer, Betty. *The Candlemaker's Companion*. Pownal, VT: Storey Publishing, 1997.

Roberts, Margaret. *Pot-Pourri Making*. Mechanicsburg, PA: Stackpole Books, 1994.

Shaudys, Phyllis. *Herbal Treasures*. Pownal, VT: Storey Publishing, 1990.

_____. *The Pleasures of Herbs*. Pownal, VT: Garden Way Publishing, 1986.

Gardening, Plants

Elpel, Thomas. *Botany in a Day*. Pony, MT: HOPS Press, 2000.

Filberti, Daphne. *"The Gift of Roses. Some Meanings for the Rose."* © Daphne Filberti, 2000-2005. RoseGathering.com. *http://www.rosegathering.com/symbols.html.*

Moldenke, Harold N. and Alma L. Moldenke . *Plants of the Bible*. New York: Dover Publications, 1986.

Webster, Helen Noyes. *"Notes on the Marjorams."* ed. Daniel J. Foley. *Herbs for Use and for Delight.* Dover Publications, 1974.

Miscellaneous Web Resources:

Gardening:

http://www.organicgardening.com/. This is Rodale's Web site and a tremendous resource.

http://www.gardenweb.com/ and *http://davesgarden.com*. On these sites, you will find hundreds of forums devoted to specific gardening topics; they also provide a gateway to the international Gardenweb sites.

http://www.herbsociety.org. Herb Society of America; if you're serious about herbs you need to join.

http://www.richters.com/. Richter's is to herb nurseries as Stonehenge is to a rubble pile. Yes, they ship worldwide—always stock mandrake seeds and sometimes even the plants.

And speaking of mandrake, you can find the autumn-blooming plant here: *http://www.arrowheadalpines.com/mno.htm*. You'll find plants you won't find anywhere else.

It will only take you a minute with Google to find a plant or herb organization—sometimes several!—devoted to your chosen plant. Do not neglect to check out your state's Department of Agriculture, which publishes a weekly or monthly broadside titled, generally, "Farmers Market Bulletin." Finally, please, please, visit and support your local independent nurseries!

Herbs, Essential Oils:

http://www.somaluna.com/. This is one of the best companies I have found. Their Information Pages alone are worth the visit. They have authentic dried mandrake root, and the Abramelin oil and incense from *Liber AL*. An excellent company throughout, recommended unreservedly!

http://www.newdirectionsaromatics.com/. Is a supplier of essential oils in truly an astounding array, and much more. It has an essential oil for relevant to every planet.

http://www.capricornslair.com/index.html. Capricorn's Lair in Ogden, Utah, has some essential oils I haven't seen elsewhere (as well as an amazing supply of seals for wax.)

A great herb company is Frontier Co-operative Herbs—*http://www.frontier-coop.com/*. Great for bulk buying

Candles:

For rolled beeswax candle materials, I recommend The Candle Maker, found online at *www.thecandlemaker.com*. They offer the all supplies you need and provide the instructions you require.

Papermaking; Bookbinding:

http://gort.ucsd.edu/preseduc/papermak.htm. This first hit I got on "Google" is a project for preschoolers, so how hard can the basic method of turning out sheets of paper be?

http://www.cs.uiowa.edu/~jones/book/. Quite a complete tutorial to book-binding, courtesy of the Department of Computer Sciences, University of Iowa.

Poppets, Corn Dollies:

Corn dollies are certainly a type of poppet; please visit *http://www.straw-craftsman.co.uk* for a complete introduction to this prehistoric craft.

Books, Online resources:

Many ancient texts are available at The Internet Classics Library. *http:// classics.mit.edu.*; likewise, *http://www.perseus.tufts.edu.* You may also find what you seek at the Gutenberg Project, *http://www.gutenberg.org*; or *http://www.sacred-texts.com*, all wonderful sites.

The Renaissance Astrology site. *http://www.renaissanceAstrology.com* offers, in addition to numerous hard-to-find texts, online courses in practical Renaissance magic.

Sepher Sephiroth [greatly expanded and revised]. © *The Magickal Review. http://www.themagickalreview.org/classics/sephiroth/dictionary.php.*

If a book you *must* have is out of print, check for it at the excellent *http://www.bookfinder.com.*

Astrology-related

Sites you should know for the lazy astrologer are *http://www.astro.com.* Visit, you'll see why. The two Planetary Hours Calculators are found at *http:// www.merchantsofatlantis.com* and *http://www.astroloji.net.*

NOTES

An Alarmingly Brief History of Herbal Magick

[1] A "sport" is an unexpected mutation in a plant's progeny, naturally occurring rather than deliberately bred.

[2] Marilynn Lawrence, "Hellenistic Astrology," Ch. 2. b, "Greek Medicine," found online at the Internet Encyclopedia of Philosophy, *http://www.iep.utm.edu.*

[3] *Cheir* is Greek for "hand," the connotation being something molded or worked by hand, commonly and in this context an herbal preparation.

[4] In some versions, Bolos succeeded in contacting the dead Ostanes after all, receiving his herbal wisdom that way. This very idea is a denial of any notion of an unbroken line of herbal magical lore. Pliny's account of this necromantic ritual is hopelessly confused. In *The Natural History*, Book XXX, 31.2, he has "Democritus," whom he consistently believes is the Greek philosopher, for Bolos, the actual operator in the ritual; and Pliny has the tomb belonging not to Ostanes, but to an entirely different mage, Dardanos.

[5] Letter, dated Nov 1st, 1932. ©1997–2006 Hermetic Order of the Golden Dawn™.

[6] It is, of course, not nearly that simple; but we have to start somewhere!

Chapter 1 — The Plants of Saturn

[1] Marsilio Ficino, *Three Books on Life*. Book 3. Chapter XXII (Tempe, AZ: Medieval and Renaissance Texts and Studies, 1998), p. 365.

[2] Aleister Crowley with Evangeline Adams, *General Principles of Astrology* (York Beach, ME: Weiser Books, 2002), p. 295.

[3] Éliphias Lévi, *Transcendental Magic* (York Beach, ME: Weiser Books, 1968), p. 252.

[4] Nicholas Culpeper, *Culpeper's Complete Herbal*. (Slough, UK: W. Foulsham & Co., Ltd., n.d.), pp. 110–111.

[5] Samuel Potter, *Therapeutics, Materia Medica and Pharmacy*. Revised by R. J. E. Scott. (York, PA: P. Blakiston's Son & Co., 1926), p. 367.

[6] Aleister Crowley, *777 and Other Qabalistic Writings of Aleister Crowley*, ed. by Israel Regardie (New York: Samuel Weiser, Inc., 1979), p. 101.

[7] Crowley, *777*, p. 100.

[8] Fred Hageneder, *The Spirit of Trees* (New York: Continuum, 2005), p. 111.

[9] Aleister Crowley, *The Book of Thoth* (New York: Samuel Weiser, Inc., 1974), p. 118.

[10] Nicholas Culpeper, *Culpeper's Complete Herbal* Slough, UK: W. Foulsham & Co., Ltd., n.d.), p. 181.

[11] Thomas Elpel, *Botany in a Day* (Pony, MT: HOPS Press, 2000). p. 43.

Chapter 2 — The Plants of Jupiter

[1] Aleister Crowley with Evangeline Adams, *The General Principles of Astrology* (Boston, MA: Weiser Books, 2006), p. 271.

[2] Crowley, 777, p. 96.

[3] Fred Hageneder. *The Meaning of Trees* (San Francisco, CA: Chronicle Books, 2005), pp 134-135.

[4] Harold N. Moldenke and Alma L. Moldenke, *Plants of the Bible* (New York: Dover Publications, 1986), p. 161.

[5] Moldenke, *Plants of the Bible*, p 160.

[6] Dion Fortune, *The Mystical Qabalah* (London & Tunbridge: Ernest Benn Ltd., 1976), p. 277.

[7] Crowley, 777, p. 100.

[8] Robert Graves, *The White Goddess* (New York: Farrar Straus and Giroux, 1981), in this particular instance, p. 177.

[9] Crowley, 777, p. 99.

[10] Readily available these days in any garden center carrying pond plants.

[11] Crowley, 777, p. 101.

Chapter 3 — The Plants of Mars

[1] Jean-Baptiste Morin, *Astrological Gallica,* Book Twenty-Two (Tempe, AZ: American Federation of Astrologers, 1994), pp. 216–217.

[2] Ellynor Barz, *Gods and Planets*, trans. Boris Matthews (Wilmette, IL: Chiron Publications, 1993), p. 40.

[3] I take this to mean that once you've chosen the day of your Mars Operation, you determine what time Scorpio will be rising that day, and time your working to happen during the first hour of Mars after that. Or you could wait for the month of Scorpio and do your work at dawn.

[4] Thomas Moore, *The Planets Within* (Hudson, NY: Lindisfarne Press, 1990), p. 186. Of course, the images can be of any type the magician desires—drawing, painting, clay sculpture—really, anything the magician can complete within that planetary hour.

[5] Hickory, tree native to North America, does not actually appear in Column XXXIX.

[6] Hageneder, *The Meaning of Trees*, pp. 175–176. But see also Stephen L. Harris and Gloria Platzner, *Classical Mythology: Images and Insights* (Mountain View, CA: Mayfield Publishing, 1995), pp. 848-850.

[7] Crowley, 777, p. 96.

[8] An odd and unlikely sounding conceit; but I never had dock growing on my property until I sowed nettle, to my continued regret. A long story. Seemed like a good idea at the time.

[9] "Traditional," maybe, to the Cypher mss. of the Secret Chiefs of the G. D., since I can't find this attribution anywhere else.

[10] Crowley, 777, p. 110. Well, perhaps "poisonous" is too strong a word, but many of the varieties have barbed tips, making them even more painful to remove. I think what is implied is "and/or."

[11] Mrs. M. Grieve, *A Modern Herbal* (Middlesex, UK: Penguin Books, 1977), p. 858.

[12] I guess she forgot about strychnine.

[13] *Potter's Therapeutics* (York, PA: P. Blakiston's Son & Co., 1926), pp. 59–60.

Chapter 4 — The Plants of the Sun

[1] Just ask a Leo.

[2] Ficino, *Three Books On Life,* Book Three, Chapter 1.70ff, p. 247.

[3] Crowley, 777, p. 97.

[4] Please, please Google "Bernini Apollo" to give yourself goosebumps!

[5] A pomegranate tree sprung from his blood. Robert Graves, *The Greek Myths. Vol. I.* (Middlesex, UK: Penguin Books, 1975), p. 78.

[6] Dionysus' history is exhaustively detailed by Graves in *The Greek Myths. Vol. 1.* Chapter 27.

[7] For a discussion comparing the motif of the sacrificed god in Freemasonry to that of Osiris slain, please see Br. Albert Pike's indispensable *Morals and Dogma of the Ancient and Accepted Scottish Rite of Freemasonry* (Richmond, VA: L.H. Jenkins, Inc., 1919), Chapter XXIV, "Prince of the Tabernacle." This book is as in-depth and solid an esoteric education as any you'll encounter.

[8] Hageneder. *The Meaning of Trees,* pp. 16, 17.

[9] Crowley, 777, p. 97.

[10] I'm here describing the species form; there are modern, garden-friendly hybrids available, with multiple blooms on the same stalk; and they are now available in a color palette from rusty reds to burnt umbers.

[11] Grieve. *A Modern Herbal,* pp. 387-388.

[12] Crowley, 777, p. 100.

[13] Dr. Wighard Strehlow and Gottfried Hertzka, *Hildegard of Bingen's Medicine* (Santa Fe, NM: Bear & Co., 1087), p. 37, quoting Hildegard's *Physica* 1134 A.

[14]Strehlow, *Hildegard of Bingen,* p. 37.

Chapter 5 — The Plants of Venus

[1] Aleister Crowley. *General Principles of Astrology* (San Francisco, CA:Weiser Books, 2006), p. 222.

[2] Jean-Baptiste Morin, *Astrologica Gallica. Book Twenty-two, Directions* (Tempe, AZ:American Federation of Astrologers, 1994), p 217.

[3] Morin, *Astrologica Gallica,* p 217.

[4] Crowley, *The Book of Thoth,* p. 79.

[5] Stephen Forrest, *The Inner Sky* (San Diego, CA: ACS Publications, (1988), p. 117.

[6] i.e., The Furies. Also called "The Eumenides" for the same reason fairies are called "The Good Folk."

[7] Graves. *The Greek Myths.* Vol. I, p. 72.

[8] Geoffrey Grigson, *The Goddess of Love* (New York: Anchor Press, 1978), p. 190.

[9] It may also be a reference to ancient games of chance, in which the favor of Venus/Aphrodite was most heartily invoked. In Roman times, tossing your dice in a "Venus"—two sixes—won you the game.

[10] Pausanius, *Descriptions of Greece*, Book 6, XXV.1. Text here is based on the following: *Pausanias Description of Greece with an English Translation by W.H.S. Jones, Litt.D., and H.A. Ormerod, M.A., in 4 Volume.* (London: William Heinemann Ltd., 1918).

[11] Grieve, *A Modern Herbal*, pp. 684–685.

[12] A contemporary rose breeder of unequalled skill.

[13] Dion Fortune, *The Mystical Qabalah* (London & Tunbridge: Ernest Benn Ltd., 1976), p. 222.

[14] Quoted by Grigson, *Goddess of Love*, p. 195.

[15] Malcolm Stuart, *Encyclopedia of Herbs and Herbalism* (London: Orbis Publishing, 1979), p. 227.

[16] Or perhaps, to Pausanius, tortoise-shaped: "Behind the portico . . . is a temple of Aphrodite. . . . The goddess in the temple they call Heavenly . . . is of ivory and gold, the work of Pheidias, and she stands with one foot upon a tortoise." *Descriptions of Greece*, XXV.1.

[17] Barbara Walker, *Woman's Dictionary of Symbols and Sacred Objects* (San Francisco, CA: Harper San Francisco, 1988), p. 449.

[18] Moldenke, *Plants of the Bible*, p. 144.

[19] J. C. Cooper, *An Illustrated Encyclopaedia of Traditional Symbols* (London: Thames & Hudson, 1987), p. 110.

[20] Pausanius, *Descriptions of Greece*, Book V, Ch. XII. 7.

[21] Grigson, *The Goddess of Love*, p. 195.

[22] Graves, *The White Goddess*, p. 262.

[23] Grieve, *A Modern Herbal*, p. 506.

[24] Pliny the Elder, *The Natural History*, Book 20, Chapter 84, is entirely devoted to the common mallow.

Chapter 6 — The Plants of Mercury

[1] Crowley and Adams, *The General Principles of Astrology*, p. 203.

[2] The ribbons, Graves writes, later became serpents. *White Goddess*, p. 66, note 3.

[3] For the whole, very funny story, please refer to *"Hymn to Hermes"* from *The Homeric Hymns*, trans. Jules Cashford (London: Penguin Books, 2003), p. 54 ff.

[4] Crowley, *The Book of Thoth*, p. 70.

[5] 777, p. 122.

[6] Aldous Huxley, *The Doors of Perception/Heaven and Hell* (New York: Harper & Row, 1990), p. 17ff.

[7] Crowley, 777, p. 97. He also refers to the plant in the Vegetable Drugs list and writes that it confers "the power of self-analysis, which is Mercurial," 777, p. 122.

[8] Fortune, *The Mystical Qabalah*, p. 249.

[9] Pliny, *Natural History*, Book 25, Chapter 10.

[10] Fortune. *The Mystical Qabalah*, p. 238; italics mine.

[11] Helen Noyes Webster, "Notes on the Marjorams," Daniel J. Foley, ed., *Herbs for Use and for Delight*. (Mineola, NY: Dover Publications, 1974), p. 81.

[12] Culpeper, *Complete Herbal*, p. 226. If it's frost-tender, you probably have a marjoram. If it takes over your garden, oregano.

[13] Grieve, *A Modern Herbal*, p. 530.

[14] And don't even get me *started* on Dittany of Crete!

[15] Crowley, 777, p. 99.

[16] Cooper, *Traditional Symbols*, p. 125.

[17] Crowley, *Book of Thoth*, p. 69; Ficino *Three Books on Life*, pp. 275, 285.

[18] Crowley, 777, p. 100.

[19] Pliny, *Natural History*, Book 26, Chapter 62.

[20] Crowley, 777, p.100.

[21] Stuart, *Herbs and Herbalism* , p. 193.

Chapter 7 — The Plants of the Moon

[1] Crowley and Adams, *The General Principles of Astrology*, p. 175.

[2] *Genesis* 5:24.

[3] Crowley, *Book of Thoth*, pp. 72–3.

[4] Crowley, *Book of Thoth*, p. 112.

[5] Fortune, *Mystical Qabalah*, pp. 252–3.

[6] Crowley, 777, p. 98, referencing Note 1 on p. 96.

[7] Crowley, in writing of the bo tree's connection with the supernal Father, claims that "its leaves suggest the phallus." (777, p. 96). Note to Mr. Crowley: With all due respect, I have grown this tree as a potted plant for several years and, except for the fact that its leaves are longer than they are wide, they have nothing of the phallus shape about them. Sometimes a peepul is only a peepul! Good, clear photographs of the mature leaves can be found at this website: *http://www.hear.org/starr/hiplants/images/thumbnails/html/ficus_religiosa.htm*.

[8] Theophrastus, *Enquiry Into Plants* trans. Arthur Hort (London: Loeb Classical Library, 1999), IX.9.1.

[9] Stuart, *Herbs and Herbalism*, p. 218.

[10] Theophrastus, *Enquiry Into Plants*, IX, viii. 7-8.

[11] Flavius Josephus, *The Wars of the Jews*, Book 7, Chapter 6, Paragraph 3, trans. William Whiston, found online at *http://www.perseus.tufts.edu/cgi-bin/ptext?lookup=J.+BJ+7.163*.

[12] Harold A. Hanson, *The Witches' Garden*, trans. Muriel Crofts (Santa Cruz, CA: Unity Press/Michael Kesend, 1978), p. 38.

[13] *http://www.arrowhead-alpines.com*; the owner writes, appropriately, that the seeds are "a bitch" to germinate.

[14] Which probably involves standing before the Throne of God. *http://www.richters.com.*

[15] Crowley, 777, p. 98.

[16] Ethan Russo, *Handbook of Psychotropic Herbs* (Binghamton, NY: Haworth Herbal Press, 2001), p. 200.

[17] Crowley, 777, p. 99.

[18] Hageneder, *The Meaning of Trees*, p. 36.

[19] The one exception is wormwood, *Artemesia absinthum*, which is given to Mars for its bitterness.

[20] Crowley, 777, p. 99

[21] Crowley, 777, p. 96.

[22] Lon Milo DuQuette, *My Life With the Spirits* (New York: Samuel Weiser Inc., 1999), p. 84, note 6.

[23] Which may have not been all that "traditional" after all. In an email to me on this subject, Dr. Robert Wang—one of the most respected scholars of the tarot, the Qabala, and the Western mystery traditions, and a close friend of Israel Regardie—wrote: "There can be no doubt that the collection in 777 ... when Mathers started this, he made it up to some extent. It has always seemed to me that when something didn't quite fit into a Western pattern, it was pushed and squeezed until it seemed to work. In other words, I think a lot of the 777 attributions are arbitrary and lack 'tradition,'" Email dated Nov. 4, 2005.

[24] Important safety note: Celtic gods really *hate* when that happens.

[25] Graves, *The White Goddess*, p. 75. The reader will recognize a variant of Cerridwen's Cauldron.

[26] Graves, *The White Goddess*, p. 182.

[27] Hilderic Friend, *Flower Lore* (Rockport, MA: Para Research, 1981), p. 314.

[28] Culpeper, *Complete Herbal*, p. 238.

[29] Gerard, *The Herbal,* p. 407.

[30] Graves, *The White Goddess*, p. 133.

[31] See Joseph Campbell, *Myths of Light: Eastern Metaphors of the Eternal* (Novato, CA: New World Library, 2003) for a wonderful expansion of this concept.

[32] Their mothers' names are equivalent.

Chapter 8 — The Plants of the Kingdom and the Four Elements

[1] Paul Simon, *Diamonds on the Soles of Her Shoes*, © Paul Simon. 1986. From his most Qabalistic album, *Graceland*.

[2] The Emerald Tablet of Hermes Trismegistus. It is elegantly parsed in Lon Milo DuQuette's *Angels, Demons & Gods of the New Millennium* (York Beach, ME: Samuel Weiser Inc., 1997), Chapter 3.

[3] DuQuette's, *Angels, Demons & Gods*, p. 62.

[4] Crowley, 777, p. 98.

[5] Robert Hand, *Horoscope Symbols* (West Chester, PA: Whitford Press, 1981), p. 186.

[6] Thanks again to *http://www.sacred-texts.com/alc/emerald.htm.*

[7] *http://www.sacred-texts.com/alc/emerald.htm.*

[8] William Blake, *The Marriage of Heaven and Hell,* plate 14, lines 12–21.

[9] Crowley, 777, p. 98.

[10] Crowley, 777, p. 98.

[11] Crowley, *Book of Thoth,* pp. 169–170.

[12] Fortune, *Mystical Qabalah,* p. 267.

[13] Steve Blamires, *Celtic Tree Mysteries* (St. Paul, MN: Llewellyn Publications, 2003), pp. 154–155.

[14] Crowley, 777, pp. 96, 97.

[15] Pausanias, *Descriptions of Greece,* 2.17.3, trans. by W.H.S. Jones (Cambridge, MA: Harvard University Press, 1918), *http://www.perseus.tufts.edu/cgi-bin/ptext?lookup=Paus.+2.17.1.*

[16] Like the menses, I suppose.

[17] Crowley, 777, p. 98.

[18] Lon Milo DuQuette, *The Chicken Qabalah of Rabbi Lamed Ben Clifford* (York Beach, ME: Weiser Books, 2001), p. 157.

[19] Crowley, 777, p. 98.

[20] Marija Gimbutas, *The Language of the Goddess* (San Francisco: Harper & Row, 1989), p. 151.

[21] Crowley, 777, p. 98.

[22] Grieve, *A Modern Herbal,* p. 651

[23] Pliny, *Natural History,* XIX. 53.

[24] Joscelyn Godwin, *Mystery Religions in the Ancient World* (San Francisco, CA: Harper & Row, 1981), pp. 33-34. The author takes as his example a 4th-century B.C.E. Apulian vase he titles "The Poppy as Mediator between Earth and Heaven."

[25] Erich Neumann, *The Great Mother* (Princeton, NJ: Princeton University Press, 1974), p. 219.

[26] Neumann, *The Great Mother,* p. 284.

[27] Dion Fortune, *Sea Priestess* (New York: Samuel Weiser, Inc., 1979), p. 214.

[28] DuQuette, *Chicken Qabalah,* p. 157.

[29] Many thanks to my teacher for pointing this out so many years ago.

[30] Reproduced on the encyclopedic Web pages of the East Lewis County Catholic Community, *http://landru.i-link-2.net/shnyves/holy_water2.htm.*

[31] Reproduced on the encyclopedic Web pages of the East Lewis County Catholic Community, *http://landru.i-link-2.net/shnyves/holy_water2.htm.*

[32] Franz Bardon, *Initiation into Hermetics* (Salt Lake City, UT: Merkur Publishing, Inc., 1999), pp. 70, 71.

[33] DuQuette, *Chicken Qabalah,* p. 44.

[34] Hand, *Horoscope Symbols,* p. 187ff.

[35] Sharing this distinction with the Tree of Knowledge, the pine, the dogwood, the elder, and the mistletoe, among, no doubt, others. The smaller ones got that way when they shrank from shame. Constantine's mother, St. Helena, found, she thought, pieces of the True Cross, and it is pine.

[36] Graves, *The White Goddess*, p. 193.

Chapter 9 — Preparing Herbs for Magick

[1] Appendix 1 of Brian Cotnoir, *The Weiser Concise Guide to Alchemy* (York Beach, ME: Weiser Books, 2005), p. 111ff. The section is devoted entirely to setting up an Alchemical laboratory. While you may not be that drawn to the demanding alchemical arts, the section "To Distill Essential Oils" may be of great interest to you!

[2] You won't find a better guide than *The Magical and Ritual Use of Perfumes* by Richard Alan Miller and Iona Miller (Rochester, VT: Destiny Books, 1990).

Chapter 10 — On Gardening

[1] Plant the variety named Poeticus or Pheasant's Eye—it's a late-blooming, very sweet-scented narcissus that is supposed to have been cultivated in ancient Greece.

Chapter 11 — The Techniques of Herbal Magick

[1] A quick Google search will turn up a number of sources for horoscope-symbol wax stamps as well as sealing wax in any color desired. For planetary seals, you may be better off inscribing the sign with a stylus, a slender pointed stick, in the still-warm wax. (You can make a stylus from the tree/plant of that planet, sign, or element.)

[2] Margaret Roberts, *Pot-Pourri Making* (Mechanicsburg, PA: Stackpole Books, 1994), p. 7.

[3] Roberts, *Pot-Pourri Making*, pp. 7–8. Also, hit the garden-section of your local home improvement store late in the fall. You'll find bags of the common bearded irises on sale for pennies. You're only going to grind them up, after all; and they're still "fresh and green" as Ms. Roberts suggests. Be bold enough to ask the manager of that section when the seasonal plant materials will go on sale. It's really ok to do so.

[4] Roberts, *Pot-Pourri Making*, p. 11.

[5] Planetary hours. Virtually any basic magical book, from Agrippa on down, will give directions for determining the planetary hours of each day, based on the sunrise and sunset times for the day in question. "Simply" divide each half (sunrise-sunset, sunset-sunrise) of the day by twelve. The "first hour" of the day will be the planetary ruler of that day. Then follow the "Chaldean system," the sequence on the Tree of Life, starting at Binah, then Chesed, and so forth. For example, for Wednesday, the first hour will be ruled by Mercury, the second by Luna, etc. I recommend that you do it a few times by hand, with a pencil and calculator, so you get the idea. However, once you know the basics, plug the phrase "planetary hour calculator" into your search engine of choice

and go from there. The Merchants of Atlantis site, *http://www.merchantsof-atlantis.com* offers one. An excellent Turkish Astrology site, *http://www.astroloji.net*, allows you to factor in your precise latitude and longitude.

[6] Roberts, *Pot-Pourri Making,* p. 18. The italics are the author's. If the ingredients are not absolutely dry, you can see how easily they'd get moldy and spoil the whole batch.

[7] Roberts, *Pot-Pourri Making,* p. 35.

[8] Ronni Lundy, *Crafts for the Spirit. 30 Beautiful Projects to Enhance Your Personal Journey* (New York: Lark Books, 2003), p. 91ff.

[9] Scott Cunningham and David Harrington, *Spell Crafts. Creating Magical Objects* (St. Paul, MN: Llewellyn Publications, 1993), Chapter 11, "Tapers of Power," p. 89ff.

[10] The instructions are given in the very highly recommended book *The Candlemaker's Companion* by Betty Oppenheimer (Pownal, VT: Storey Publishing, 1997), p. 19ff.

[11] Ms. Oppenheimer recommends a warm room, a hairdryer, or the sheets on thin cardboard on top of a heating pad set on "low" and watched like a hawk. *Candelmaker's Companion,* p. 57.

[12] You will find the original page at *http://www.angelfire.com/realm/white_witch.*

[13] The plain text is ©White Witch 2001; the italics are my own additions.

[14] See Resources and Bibliography on p. 114 for information on Phyllis Shaudy's *Herbal Treasures.* Instuctions for drying whole flower heads will be found in her book on p. 137ff.

[15] Laura C. Martin, *The Art and Craft of Pounding Flowers* (Mt. Kisco, NY: QVC Publishing, 2001).

Chapter 12 — Franz Bardon and Herbal Magick

[1] Bardon, *Initiation into Hermetics,* p. 101ff, and for more advanced meditations, p. 231ff.

[2] A guess here, based on Bardon's earlier invocation of the Law of Signatures, is that he intuited his herbs. His present-day students will point out how much esoteric knowledge Bardon brought through from his past lives.

To Our Readers

THE WEISER CONCISE GUIDES

A series of books, edited by James and Nancy Wasserman, designed to provide clear and accurate introductions to the most important disciplines of the Western Esoteric Tradition. Each book is written by a knowledgeable expert in the field under discussion. Broad overviews of each topic are augmented by explicit instructions for beginning and enhancing one's practice. Each author discusses the relevance of the subject matter at hand to the personal life of the reader. Why is this an important topic? What will it bring to my life? Bibliographies of the best work in each field are provided, allowing the reader to continue his or her studies with the most discerning authorities.

Alchemy
BRIAN COTNOIR

A guide to the theory and practice of alchemy with instructions on actually performing the alchemical work and setting up a laboratory for further experimentation. Illuminates both the spiritual and physical aspects of this ancient science and art.

Yoga for Magick
NANCY WASSERMAN

A guide to the theory and practice of yoga and meditation specifically designed for the practioner of Western disciplines such as Magick, Wicca, Paganism, and Qabalah. Includes extensive information on diet and suggestions for pursuing a healthy lifestyle.

Check out:

www.redwheelweiser.com

or

www.studio31.com

for future titles and more information on each book in this series.